NURSING THE DYING

NURSING THE DYING

DAVID FIELD

Lecturer in Department of Sociology
and Medical School, University of Leicester

TAVISTOCK/ROUTLEDGE

First published 1989
by Routledge
11 New Fetter Lane, London EC4P 4EE
29 West 35th Street, New York, NY 10001

© 1989 David Field

Set in 10/12 Baskerville by
Mayhew Typesetting, Bristol
and printed in Great Britain by
Mackays of Chatham PLC, Chatham, Kent

British Library Cataloguing in Publication Data

Field, David
Nursing the dying.
1. Terminally ill patients. Home care
I. Title
610.73′61

ISBN 0-415-01053-5
ISBN 0-415-01054-3 (pbk)

Contents

Acknowledgements   vii

PART ONE   PRELIMINARIES

1   Introduction   3
*General background; Attitudes towards death and dying;
Disclosure of terminal prognoses; Plan of the book*

2   Preliminary considerations   12
*The organization of nursing; Hospitals as organizations; The
organization of hospitals and care of the dying; Hospice care;
Summary*

PART TWO   NURSING THE DYING

3   'A silent conspiracy': nursing terminally ill cancer
patients on an acute surgical ward   35
*The ward; The patient sample; Recognizing impending death;
Relationships on the ward; Communication on the ward;
Summary*

4   'We didn't want him to die on his own': nursing
dying patients on a general medical ward   46
*The ward; Aspects of dying; Awareness contexts; Emotional
involvement; Dealing with relatives; The organization of work
and nursing the dying*

5 'Death is no failure': nursing the terminally ill on a
   coronary care unit   63
   *The unit; Working on the unit; Death on the unit; Coping
   with death; Communication with dying patients; Emotional
   involvement; Dealing with relatives; Summary*

6 'I never interfere with what they want': nursing
   terminally ill people at home   92
   *Differences between hospital and community nursing; Nursing
   people dying at home; Awareness, communication, and the
   nurse's role; Concluding comments*

PART THREE   DISCUSSION

7 The organization of nursing work and nursing people
   who are dying   113
   *Work settings; Work organization; Doctor – nurse relationships;
   The role of the ward sister; Disclosure norms; Nurses'
   attitudes and predispositions; Communication skills; Patient
   contact; Emotional involvement; Some recommendations;
   Summary*

8 Postscript: some wider considerations   139
   *Changing attitudes towards the care of the dying; The impact
   of AIDS; Problems within nursing; Changes in the NHS;
   Powerless patients*

   Methodological appendix   150
   *Theoretical background; The sample; Data collection and
   analysis; General problems of the interview method*

   References   161

   Index   171

Acknowledgements

This book has had a long gestation period and so there are many people to thank for their help and support.

My first thanks go to the nurses who talked to me about their experiences and attitudes. Without them quite evidently this book would not appear. I trust they recognize it as a faithful account.

Throughout the time of the project David Ashton offered help, encouragement, criticism, and a listening ear for my problems; he also read and commented upon all of the draft chapters of the thesis upon which this book is based. In the later stages Nicky James provided invaluable comments, suggestions, and criticisms. Bryan Turner, the reader for Routledge, was very helpful in his criticisms and suggestions for improvement of the original manuscript. Judith Smith provided secretarial support over and beyond the mere bounds of duty, especially during the transcription of the interview transcripts. Mary Knight was the participant observer for the study reported in Chapter three. I thank all of them for their important contributions towards this final product.

A number of other people also provided material and psychological help and encouragement: Gerry Bowman, Alan Davis, Ian Hankinson, Kevin Howells, Mike Kelly, Susan Kendall, Colin Rees, and Ivan Waddington, and many others who commented helpfully on drafts and presentations of various chapters. I am especially grateful to members of the Medical Sociology Group of the British Sociological Association who provided me with my annual 'fix' of professional support and trips to the disco floor. I thank all these people for their help.

Finally I thank the *Journal of Advanced Nursing* for allowing me to use articles published in that journal as the basis for Chapters three and four.

vii

Part One

PRELIMINARIES

The availability of good care tends to vary inversely with the number of people suffering from a condition. And we all die.
Cartwright, Hockey, and Anderson, *Life Before Death*

Chapter One

Introduction

It has often been noted that death is the only certainty in life, yet in our society we seem to handle death and dying poorly. Cartwright *et al.*, in their survey of the last year of life of a national sample of those who had died, concluded that the 'inverse care law' applies in death as in life: '[t]he availability of good care tends to vary inversely with the number of people suffering from a condition. And we all die' (1973:228). Two important factors underpinning this parlous situation are prevailing attitudes towards death and dying, especially those towards disclosure of a terminal prognosis to those people who are dying, and the organization of the care of dying people in our society. Modern attitudes towards death and dying are marked by apprehension, fear, and avoidance, and these attitudes interact with the increased institutionalization of the care of those dying in hospitals, where disclosure of a terminal prognosis is unusual. Within hospitals most of the work of caring for dying people falls to nurses. This book looks at the factors which affect such nursing work and is based upon nurses' accounts of nursing dying people.

GENERAL BACKGROUND

The book has its origins in the author's teaching experiences with medical and nursing students. Most of the literature about death and dying in modern societies which was used in teaching about this topic was drawn from the United States, and mainly focused upon doctors. Was it legitimate, therefore, to generalize from such material to the problems of nursing dying people in modern Britain? Contemporary US and British societies share some common features, but there are significant differences in values and attitudes, and their organization of health care is vastly different (Hiatt 1987; Rodwin 1984; Roemer 1977; Stacey 1985). Did the differences outweigh the similarities in shaping nurses' experiences of and responses to nursing dying people? The research which forms the core of this book was intended to throw some light on the question of whether US research findings could be generalized to the British situation, a question which is answered in the affirmative. It does seem that the problems experienced by British and US nurses in nursing people who are dying are very similar, and that each society can learn from the research and attempted solutions found in the other.

The main influence upon this research was the work which was conducted in the United States by Glaser and Strauss and their co-workers (Glaser and Strauss 1965, 1968; Quint 1967). This is reviewed in the next chapter. Their research emphasized the centrality of the patterns of communication between caregivers and dying people for the ways in which death and dying were handled, and for the ways in which all participants experienced the situation. In particular they emphasized that people's awareness of dying was important to the way in which dying was experienced, and they documented the tendency for caregivers to attempt to keep people who are dying from becoming aware that they are terminally ill. Other writers, especially Kubler-Ross (1970, 1975) and those from the hospice tradition have subsequently emphasized the disadvantages of caregivers attempting to maintain such a 'conspiracy of silence' in their communication with dying people. The starting point for this book was a concern with nurses communication with patients who were dying. The book is about the interplay between nurses' attitudes towards dying people, and the social organization of the situations within which they perform such nursing work. It therefore describes such attitudes and attempts to specify those features of the organization of nursing work which constrain, facilitate, and shape interactions with dying people, and hence influence attitudes and behaviour towards them.

ATTITUDES TOWARDS DEATH AND DYING

There is good reason to believe that there is a relationship between the attitudes held towards death and dying by caregivers and the psycho-social experiences and well-being of people who are dying. The difficulties met by terminally ill people may be exacerbated by the failure of doctors and nurses to deal adequately with their own reactions to death and dying. In particular the lack of knowledge about the nature of their condition and the social isolation of many terminally ill patients are likely to be, at least in part, a product of the difficulties which hospital staff have in discussing and dealing with death and dying (Backer *et al.* 1982; Charles-Edwards 1983; Glaser and Strauss 1965, 1968; Lowenberg 1976; Munn 1983; Quint 1967; Redding 1980; Sudnow 1967). Nurses and doctors are subject to experiences and beliefs similar to those of the rest of society, and so could be expected to hold attitudes and beliefs towards death and dying broadly resembling those of the general population. In making sense of their experiences with people who are dying nurses will draw upon such attitudes and beliefs. However, they have more frequent and sustained contact with death and dying than do most other members of our society, and the nature of such contact can be intense and highly stressful (Charles-Edwards 1983; Gow 1982; Vachon 1987).

In his ground-breaking discussion of 'Death and social structure' Blauner (1966) argued that death is less pervasive and central in modern societies than in non-modern societies, and linked this firmly to changes in demographic structure resulting from changing patterns of mortality. Mainly as a result of low rates of mortality in the early years of life, a significant proportion of the population of a modern industrial society such as Britain is beyond working age. In 1984 15 per cent of the British population was over the age of 65, and 6.4 per cent over the age of 75 (Office of Population Censuses and Surveys 1986b: Table 1.1). Death in our society now mainly occurs among these age groups, with the result that 'as death . . . becomes increasingly a phenomenon of the old, who are usually retired from work and finished with their parental responsibilities, mortality in modern society rarely interrupts the business of life' (Blauner 1966:379). Such societies have also, according to Blauner, 'bureaucratized death' by making hospitals, funeral organizations, and the like primarily responsible for its management. Thus it can be largely ignored by the general population, although the lack of funeral and mourning rituals may make it harder for the bereaved to cope with their loss. This argument has been largely accepted, with many writers suggesting that members of modern western societies are less accepting and more apprehensive of death than were people in previous eras because individually they have less exposure to death and dying. As Elias puts it, psychologically people can keep death at a distance because 'it is easier in the normal course of life to forget death' (1985:8). Elias argues that modern western societies are characterized by a high degree of individualization, and that their members experience themselves as unique and separate beings rather than as members of tightly knit groups in which their individuality is submerged. Because death is no longer surrounded and made sense of by the rituals of departure of earlier times – such as the elaborate mourning customs of Victorian Britain – individuals have to make sense of death and dying on their own, rather than drawing upon the collective wisdom of the group. The infrequency of death, individuation, and the absence of shared meanings and rituals about death and dying combine to make them unfamiliar and feared conditions.

More contentiously some writers have taken the argument a step further and argued that these societies are 'death denying' and 'death avoiding'. In his influential book Gorer (1965) suggested that death had become a taboo topic in the twentieth century, replacing sex as the area which it was forbidden to discuss or mention. Similarly, Aries asserts, 'The old attitude in which death was both familiar and near, evoking no great fear or awe, offers too marked a contrast to ours where death is so frightful that we dare not utter its name' (1974:13). However, there is no consensus on the validity of this view, and it seems hard to sustain (Kellehear 1984). For example, a national US survey 'found that most people of all ages held non-threatening images of death' (Riley 1983). Since the mid-1960s death and dying have become if not popular topics at least the subjects of debate, discussion, and research. In 1979 Simpson reported that there were more than 750 books on the general topic, and his revised bibliography considers 1700 books currently in print (Simpson 1979, 1987). Discussion of death and dying is certainly not restricted to a limited group of practitioners and researchers, as any cursory survey of the mass media will attest.

In Britain a study of the views of older Aberdonians (Williams 1989) seems to offer a more satisfactory picture of the attitudes towards death and dying in our society. Williams reported that four coherent patterns could be seen in his respondents in their thinking about death. The most common pattern was that of 'disregarded death'. This is similar to the picture described by Blauner and others, and included a preference for a quick death which the respondent was unaware of, although this was often seen as difficult for the bereaved to cope with. Also common was a pattern of attitudes similar to those attributed by Aries and Elias to an earlier period of European history and which Williams calls 'ritual death'. Here respondents believed that the dying person should be prepared for his or her death, be aware of it, and have had the opportunity to make farewells to relatives and friends. An important feature of the study is the complexity of the attitudes uncovered. Williams suggests that different 'strata' of attitudes are evident, with an emerging pattern of 'controlled dying' focusing around the core ideas of an aware terminally ill person who might wish to have the option of euthanasia. Attitudes were not necessarily clear-cut, and people often held what they recognized to be conflicting views, for example that a quick death was desirable and that death should occur after saying goodbye to the family. Generally speaking the Aberdeen study supports the view that people do not wish to know about their impending death, but does not necessarily support the view that death is highly feared and avoided. The latter may be a result of the age of the sample, as other research consistently reports that elderly people are more accepting and less fearful of death than younger people.

DISCLOSURE OF TERMINAL PROGNOSES

Normally the decision whether or not to disclose 'bad news', especially a terminal prognosis, is controlled by doctors. Until recently doctors and other hospital staff did not normally inform patients that they were dying. It seems between 70 and 90 per cent of physicians preferred not to inform patients of their impending death (Cartwright et al. 1973; Duff and Hollingshead 1968; Fitts and Radvin 1953; Gilbertsen and Wangensteen 1961; McIntosh 1977; Oken 1961; Ward 1974a, 1974b). Nurses have been reported to show a similar reluctance to disclose such information (Bond 1983; Charles-Edwards 1983; McIntoch 1977; Simpson 1975). Failure to inform dying patients that they are dying persists for a number of reasons. There may be genuine uncertainty with regard to both outcome and/or the time of death. Some doctors and nurses claim that non-disclosure protects the patient from depression and anxiety. It also protects hospital staff from becoming too closely implicated in the patients' dying and so they can maintain the pretence of 'everything as normal' and not get involved in the personal aspects of handling the death. In a similar way it may be thought to 'protect' or 'make things easier for' the family. Finally, the work routines of the ward or unit may be disrupted by disclosure of impending death and the resulting necessity for staff to spend time coping with the psychological problems of dying patients. Whatever the reasons it seems that it was, and in many British hospitals still is, the general practice to conceal the fact of their impending death from dying patients.

An influential body of opinion (Saunders 1959, 1978; Saunders et al. 1981; Hinton 1972; Kubler-Ross 1970, 1975) holds that dying patients should be informed of their terminal condition for both moral and 'practical management' reasons, and there is a growing body of evidence to suggest that there has been a move within medicine and nursing towards greater openness with dying patients than existed a decade or so ago (Bowling and Cartwright 1982; Carey and Posavic 1978; Greenwald and Nevitt 1982; Novack et al. 1979; Rea et al. 1975). There are a number of reasons adduced in favour of a policy of disclosure of their terminal prognosis to people who are dying. It is argued that disclosure resolves the problems of 'forced pretence' and patient suspicion by allowing open discussion between patient, staff, and families. It thus obviates the problem of patient mistrust in the face of 'a conspiracy of silence', and reduces the loneliness and isolation of the patient which would otherwise result from the denials of others that anything is wrong, coupled with their withdrawal from the dying patient. It is also claimed that non-disclosure of terminal prognosis to the suspicious patient, far from diminishing anxiety, actually increases it, whereas disclosure of prognosis decreases anxiety and ultimately depression. The lack of communication between caregivers and dying patients in situations of non-disclosure can directly result in patients receiving inadequate pain relief and attention to their physical needs. Physical and mental pain are closely related, and openness, by alleviating anxiety, seems to have a positive effect on the management of distressing physical symptoms, especially pain. Further, patients who are aware of their impending death may put their practical affairs in order, make their goodbyes, and 'finish off their lives' symbolically.

There seem to be three good reasons for not withholding the disclosure of terminal prognosis from a dying person. First, most dying patients become aware that they are dying even if this information is withheld from them (Carey and Posavic 1978; Cartwright *et al.* 1973; Glaser and Strauss 1965, 1968; Hinton 1972; Kubler-Ross 1970; Witzel 1975). Second, it is consistently reported that when asked, a substantial majority of people indicate that they would want to know if they were dying (Kelly and Friesen 1950; Aitken-Swan and Easson 1959; Cappon 1959; Gilbertsen and Wangensteen 1961). Third, those who do not wish to know of their impending death seem 'not to hear' such news (Kubler-Ross 1970). The 'conventional wisdom' which seems to be developing within medicine and nursing is that openness and honesty are important aids to assisting the terminally ill with their dying, and that such openness is beneficial for staff by easing stress. However, it is acknowledged that *when* and *how* to disclose the bad news remains problematic.

PLAN OF THE BOOK

Most deaths in our society occur in hospitals or other institutions for the care of the sick. The main group of people caring for people who are dying in these institutions are nurses. This book looks at nursing dying people as seen from the perspective of nurses, and mainly focuses upon hospital nurses dealing with adult patients. The focus is further narrowed in that the concern is with social and psychological aspects of nursing those who are dying and not with the 'practical nursing work' which is involved. In particular, as has already been noted, the book is concerned with the interplay between nurses' attitudes, especially those related to communication with dying patients and to their emotional involvement with such patients, and organizational features of nursing work which affect the care of dying people. The latter is vital for, as Vachon so succinctly expresses it, 'Dying patients are not the real problem.' The 'real problems' lie in the organization of the work environment, and so may prove intractable to solution by the individual action of nurses (Vachon 1987).

In order to investigate the influence of the organization of work upon the care of dying people, nurses working in three different settings were interviewed: nurses at a general medical ward and a coronary care unit at Midland General Hospital, where an acute surgical ward had previously been studied, and community nurses. In all of these settings the nurses were dealing with adult patients, and so this book does not look at problems of nursing infants or children who are dying. Some extracts from the transcribed interviews are slightly edited, and this is indicated thus: (. . .). To preserve confidentiality nurses are indicated by an arbitrarily assigned letter which is prefixed by an indication of their status: C = charge nurse or sister; E = enrolled nurse; P = pupil nurse; R = registered nurse; S = student nurse. The researcher is referred to as DF. Further details of the methods used are found in the Appendix. It should be said at the outset that the medical ward and coronary care unit appear to be exceptional, and provide evidence of the possibility of good nursing care of people dying in our hospitals. This is not to say that the nurses on these units were themselves exceptional but that they were enabled by the organization of their work to implement their ideals of nursing patients who were dying, something which a number of them said they were unable to do in other settings where they had worked.

The next chapter serves to place the research reported in Chapters three through six in the context of the relevant research about hospitals and the handling of death in them. It also considers the impact of the hospice movement upon the care of the dying, and provides a general discussion of nursing as an occupation. Chapter three briefly reports a participant observation study of an acute surgical ward at Midland General Hospital. Chapter four looks at nurses' accounts of nursing dying patients on a general medical ward, Chapter five at a coronary care unit, and Chapter six at nursing people dying in the community. The next chapter discusses the organization of nursing work and its impact upon the nursing of dying people, drawing upon the research presented in these chapters and by others, and suggests possible ways of improving such work. The final chapter provides a brief overview of more general matters relating to the nursing care of people dying in our society. The attempt has been made to avoid the sexist use of language, but where to do so would have been unduly clumsy nurses are generically referred to as female, since this reflects the preponderance of females in the occupation and in the research reported in Chapters three through six.

Chapter Two

Preliminary considerations

Nursing dying people is work or, to use James's (1986) evocative term, 'carework'. This chapter therefore provides an orienting discussion of the two main constraints upon such work: hospital organizations and the way in which nursing is organized. The chapter begins by looking at the organization of nursing and the effects of this upon nursing care of dying people. It then goes on to discuss the organization of hospitals and the general consequences of such organizational arrangements for the care of dying patients. This is followed by a more detailed look at the care of those dying in hospitals by way of a discussion of key studies, and in particular a review of material bearing upon communication, awareness, and disclosure of dying in hospitals. The hospice movement has had an important impact upon the care of those who are dying, and so this is discussed in the final section of the chapter.

THE ORGANIZATION OF NURSING

The way in which the nursing profession is organized has a bearing on the nursing care of dying patients. Of particular salience are patterns of recruitment, training, and nursing turnover, and the organization of nursing work. A review of the development of nursing will not be attempted here, but some salient features can be traced back to at least the Victorian era and the Nightingale reforms of the training and organization of nursing (Abel-Smith 1960; Bullough and Bullough 1979; Davies 1981; Ehrenreich and English 1974; Freidson 1970; Gamarnikow 1978). These features are the female basis of nursing, its subordination to medicine, its primary location within hospitals, its hierarchical organization, and the lack of autonomy afforded to nurses.

The key feature of nursing as an occupation is its definition in relation to the medical profession as a subordinate and ancillary activity. This largely stems from the concentration of nursing work in the hospital, where the parameters of nursing activity are controlled largely by other groups within the hospital hierarchy, especially doctors. This feature dates from the Victorian era and Nightingale's definition of nursing work, which Freidson summarizes as follows: 'All nursing work flowed from the doctor's orders, and thus nursing became part of doctor's work, a technical trade rather than a "natural" practice of femininity or a part of the exercise of charitable impulses. Nursing was thus defined as a subordinate part of the technical division of labour surrounding medicine' (1970:61). This view highlights the emphasis on the 'technical' aspect of nursing as an occupation while downplaying the extent to which the occupation rests upon 'natural' female skills and attributes. Both aspects are relevant to an understanding of contemporary nursing, and debate continues over their relative importance, with a strong drive from the nursing leadership to emphasize and enhance the technical and 'professional' basis of nursing.

Nurses today are recruited predominantly from among young females (United Kingdom Central Council 1986), most of whom, it seems, enter nursing with a conception of nursing as a caring occupation – what Schulman called the 'mother surrogate' role (Schulman 1972; Moloney 1986). Ten per cent of nurses are now males, but these are found primarily in psychiatric nursing, and in administrative positions within the nursing hierarchy (Salvage 1985; Stacey 1985). This pattern of recruitment and orientation suggests that – despite the number of male nurses – nursing can be usefully seen as a 'gendered job'. That is, one 'which capitalizes on the skills women have by virtue of having lived their lives as women . . . these skills go unacknowledged and unrewarded, . . . where they are seen at all, they are seen as qualities which attach to a particular woman or to women as a group' (Davies and Rosser 1986:109). The particular skill which nursing as a gendered job draws upon is that of caring (Graham 1983; James 1986). Graham defines caring as 'encompassing that range of human experiences which have to do with feeling concern

13

for, and taking charge of, the well-being of others' (1983:13). It demands both labour and love, and in our society is firmly linked to the female role, both in terms of women's conceptions of themselves and in terms of the expectations of others. Women take care of men, children, the elderly, and the sick as part of an often invisible network of social and economic relationships which keep society functioning. Nursing extends this activity from the unpaid to the paid sector.

Feminist writers such as Graham (1983) thus suggest that the technical work of nursing is suffused with and depends upon presumed 'natural' female practices of care, and that the caring function is transferred from the domestic realm into nursing work but without fundamentally altering either the nature of caring work or the social relationships surrounding it. Gamarnikow (1978) argues that it is not simply that nursing occupies a sub-ordinate position to medicine, but that this reflects the power relationships between men and women in the wider society. She uses the analogy of the family to describe the relationship between doctors (patriarchal fathers), nurses (subordinate mothers), and patients (children to be cared for). During the Victorian era, 'the moral traits of the "good nurse" were evidently seen within the profession itself as identical with the characteristics desirable in a "good woman"' (Gamarnikow 1978:98), a situation which still seems to apply today. Also in that time, she argues, 'many aspects of the nurses' work became identifiable with domestic labour' (1978:98). Game and Pringle (1983) also use the analogy of the family, arguing further that doctor–nurse relationships are shaped by highly sexualized power relations. The doctor–nurse relationship of superordination/subordination thus reflects an enduring pattern of male–female relationships within western society, and is not based simply on functionally differentiated roles and tasks within health-care work (Quint 1967).

The attempts to 'professionalize' nursing by rooting it in such ideas of holistic care as are embodied in the nursing process (Crow and Kratz 1977; Henderson 1969) seem to represent a fusion of the 'traditional' and 'technical/professional' aspects of nursing around the (idealized) traditional nurturant and caring role of the nurse. Despite this, the nursing process is often viewed with suspicion and hostility by nurses in the wards, and is not implemented wholeheartedly (Melia 1987; Salvage 1985). At a more general level, Salvage claims that 'professionalization' is a narrow, interest-centred strategy pursued by the nursing elite which ignores the interests of the rank-and-file nurses and its effects upon such nurses and patients. Moloney (1986) makes a similar point with reference to the nursing profession in the United States. Armstrong (1983) claims that it is only very recently that the notion of care in nursing has been extended beyond the biological to include psychological factors and communication in the emphasis upon holistic patient care. Whatever the exact truth of these analyses of the development and function of 'caring' in nursing, it is currently seen as central to the nursing role and training schools' attempt to provide a philosophy and practice of care for their trainees.

The fact that most nurses are female does appear to contribute significantly to the continuation of the subordinate position of the nurse in the hospital hierarchy despite general changes towards greater equality elsewhere (Game and Pringle 1983; Rosenthal *et al.* 1980), and may contribute to the already noted reluctance of nurses to go against 'doctor's orders' to withhold terminal prognosis from patients. While the physiological, psychological, and social *care* – as distinct from the therapeutic cure or treatment – of the patient is primarily the province of the nursing staff, such care is at least nominally under the control of the doctor. Doctors can and do impose restrictions on the care offered by nurses to patients (e.g. Quint 1967). (The absence of the *patient* from this description should be noted: patients rarely figure as actors in the decisions which are made about and for them, even though their relatives may become involved.) Two features of the doctor–nurse relationship in particular seem to be crucial to the care of patients who are dying. First, it is the doctor who decides whether 'active' curative treatment aimed at eliminating or controlling the disease process – sometimes at the price of unpleasant 'side effects' – shall be continued as the main focus of attention, or whether it should be replaced by an emphasis on the assessment and control of symptoms in 'palliative' terminal care. While such decisions may be made in discussion with nurses it is the doctor who has the final say, and who legitimates entry to the dying 'career'. Second, the doctor controls the information which nurses are allowed to give to patients and to relatives about diagnosis and prognosis. Nurses may be forbidden to reveal that a patient is dying, even if they consider that such information should be given. It is not being suggested that relations between doctors and nurses are exclusively hierarchical and formal, as there may be much discussion and negotiation between them about patient care, especially when a 'team' has been together for a long time.

The recruitment of young females has consequences for nursing turnover. Turnover, which is high, is partly explicable by the pattern of nurses leaving work to have and raise families (Hockey 1976), and partly by low pay – a characteristic of predominantly female occupations (Department of Employment 1985; Redfern 1981; Salvage 1985; Webb 1982). One of the disadvantages nurses face in this respect is that as they comprise over 40 per cent of the National Health Service's wages and salaries bill, the government of the day has a vested interest in restricting their pay rises. Nurses have not been renowned for their militancy in pursuit of better pay and conditions, usually placing concerns for 'patient care' before industrial action, and the Royal College of Nurses has a 'no strike policy'. Women are typically underrepresented by trades unions, but in recent years British nurses have been joining the two health workers' unions COHSE and NUPE in larger numbers, and are showing more militancy in their search for better pay and conditions (Salvage 1985), throughout most participation in the industrial unrest in the NHS in the early part of 1988. The nature of nurse training may be another factor leading to high rates of turnover. As Salvage (1985) comments, in certain fundamental ways training seems to have altered very little, and is still based upon the primacy of cheap labour, with educational requirements subordinated to service needs, and the rights of students usually ignored. The proposals fundamentally to change this situation by introducing a system emphasizing the primacy of the educational requirements of trainees while they are on the wards (Royal College of Nursing 1986; United Kingdom Central Council 1986) could change this situation. However, continuing recruitment and turnover problems are likely, and under such circumstances nursing may become more dependent upon untrained nursing auxiliaries – a group already providing a large amount of the care of dying patients – despite efforts to decrease the importance of this category.

The organization of nurse training has contributed to the inability of nurses fully to control their work partly by its effect on the organization of nursing work on the wards, and partly by the psychological effects it has on students and pupils. This has been well described by Melia (1984, 1987), among others, who points up the contradictions between the training school and ward experiences of the trainees. The discrepancy between the school-based 'professional' and the ward-based 'traditional' strands in nursing is marked (Habenstein and Christ 1955; Moloney 1986), and the view of nursing found in the two locations is very different. Nursing schools are likely to emphasize the professional role of the nurse and to see social and emotional problems as part of the legitimate area of nursing concern, and to transmit a view of individualized or 'whole person care' as embodied in the use of the 'nursing process' (Henderson 1969; Crow and Kratz 1977). By contrast, senior hospital nurses are more likely to emphasize a management, 'task-oriented' approach to nursing (Melia 1987; Pembrey 1980; Redfern 1981; Runciman 1983), and on most wards trainees are seen as essentially another pair of hands (Clarke 1978), and are given the routine day-to-day work which has to be done. They are not, it seems, systematically trained to assume responsibility, to take decisions about the care of individual patients, or to talk to patients. The messages given in training school are not usually reinforced and supported on the wards (Bendall 1976; Melia 1987; Simpson 1980).

With specific reference to nurse education about death and dying, Game and Pringle (1983) claim that the subject of death 'was carefully avoided in training' until recently. The results of a 1984 survey of British nursing schools (Field 1986) suggests that this is no longer the case, and that it is a topic receiving serious attention in these schools. Studies from the United States report more favourable, less fearful, and less avoiding attitudes towards death and dying as a result of death education (Bugen 1980; Leviton 1978–9; Miles 1980; Murray 1974; Watts 1977). However, in Britain a survey by Birch (1983) presents a generally unsatisfactory picture of teaching about death and bereavement in our nursing schools, and many of Field's respondents expressed reservations about the efficacy of their teaching even though there was a generally positive view of the impact of their teaching upon trainees. The main reservations expressed related to the lack of correspondence between the school situation and the trainees' experiences on the wards. It does seem that training for the

17

nursing of dying patients is still inadequate, especially with reference to psycho-social factors. For example Wilkes reports that half the junior doctors and nurses he interviewed thought their training in terminal care was inadequate (1984). Yet the care of people who are dying in hospitals often devolves to nursing auxiliaries and pupil and student nurses who are unskilled, unprepared, and often unsupported by their more experienced colleagues (Knight and Field 1981; Quint 1967). Melia's apt description of the trainee as 'nursing in the dark' seems to have particular weight where dying patients are concerned.

The importance of further training as a means to career advancement is another factor leading to high rates of turnover of nurses on hospital wards (Melia 1987). This pattern of recruitment and high rates of turnover means that most nurses will have had little, if any, direct experience of death and dying, especially during the early years of their nursing career. For example Simpson (1975), in his study of student nurses in London, found that only 12 per cent had experienced a death in their family, and that 35 per cent had never witnessed death, not even during their training. This lack of general and death-related experience creates difficulties for the nurses in their work with patients who are dying (Charles-Edwards 1983). It must also, one presumes, have profound effects upon their care, and upon the experience of dying for the terminally ill and their relatives.

HOSPITALS AS ORGANIZATIONS

One of the achievements of the NHS has been the transformation of the decaying, disorganized, understaffed, uncoordinated, and near bankrupt set of hospitals it inherited from local and municipal authorities into a well-organized and coordinated service. Of particular relevance here was the 1962 Hospital Plan for England and Wales, which led to the establishment of the district general hospital of 600 to 800 beds as the core unit in the hospital sector (Allsop 1984). Such a hospital provided the study site for the research reported in the next three chapters. These hospitals were intended to provide an extensive range of services (which they do) and to replace smaller, inefficient hospitals (an element partially reversed in the 1970s). From 1959 to 1980 the number of NHS hospitals decreased by a quarter, although at the same time the number of 250–1,000-bed hospitals doubled (Fry *et al.* 1984). Alongside the building and refurbishing of general hospitals there has been a change in the pattern of hospital use. The number of hospital beds has declined while the number of patients treated per bed has increased. For example from 1961 to 1980 the number of patients treated per bed during a year doubled from 15.4 to 31. Each year 12 per cent of the British population is admitted to hospital with an average length of stay of eight days – a reduction of 30 per cent in the duration of stay since 1970 (Fry *et al.* 1984). The 1962 hospital plan reinforced the dominance of the hospital sector within the NHS, a dominance reflected in the allocation of over 60 per cent of the NHS budget to the hospital sector in every year since 1960, and the ever increasing number of patients and conditions treated in our hospitals. One element within this trend has been the steady shift from a pattern of people dying at home to that of people dying in hospital.

In England and Wales in 1984 over 62 per cent of all deaths occurred in hospitals or other institutions for the care of the sick, and nearly another 6 per cent of all deaths took place in other institutions (Office of Population Censuses and Surveys 1986a). Nearly 5.5 per cent of all hospital admissions in England in 1984 were 'discharged dead' (Government Statistical Services 1986). Cartwright *et al.* (1973) estimated that nearly a third of all hospital beds were occupied by patients who were dying, or who would die within the year. While the experience of dying patients and their relatives is unique and problematic, for hospital staff care of the dying is part of their work. The ways in which staff define and perform such work has an important, if not crucial, effect on the experience of dying for patients and their relatives. Such definitions and performance are themselves shaped in various ways by the organizational demands and routines of hospital life, and by 'external factors' such as budget allocations to hospitals for staff and equipment, which will influence these organizational arrangements. The two groups of hospital staff most directly concerned with such work are nurses and doctors, with the everyday care and close contact with dying patients falling to the former.

Hospitals are organizations characterized by a number of sometimes competing goals and an increasingly complex division of labour (Alexander 1984; Freidson 1963, 1970; Mauksch 1966,

1975; Morgan *et al.* 1985:141–51; Perrow 1965; Strauss *et al.* 1985; Tuckett 1976). The research of Strauss *et al.* makes the complexity of hospital work abundantly evident. They point out that modern hospital care involves a plethora of staff, and that different staff will be more or less responsible for different types of work. Staffing levels, coordination of activities between staff, and disputes between staff over work priorities and performance will obviously affect patient care. They further note that 'hospitals are quite decentralised in terms of their ward functioning and work' (p. 75), although to some extent such autonomy is limited by the dependence of wards and units on other parts of the hospital for resources and services. Hospitals can thus be seen as comprising 'multiple work sites' with little central coordination or control over these various 'workshops'. Not only are the work sites different from each other in terms of their organizational and clinical work, but within each a variety of work tasks must be performed and coordinated. Strauss *et al.* identify and discuss a number of types of work done by nurses, doctors, and other staff.

With the trend towards more complex medical technology and dependence upon machines in medical care, looking after and maintaining these machines ('machine work') is an increasingly important aspect of nursing work. One of the pressures in nursing work is to develop its medico-technical aspect, as reflected in the recommendation of the UKCC's *Project 2000* to develop a range of clinical specialist practitioners (United Kingdom Central Council 1986:40–2). Specialist nurses can already be found in the special care units, where their work is focused around connecting machines to patients and monitoring their performance. One consequence of such work is that nurses may become less concerned with patient performance and more concerned with machine performance. 'Safety work' is an essential part of nursing in all settings. 'Comfort work' is also ubiquitous, but may take a lesser role in the face of other tasks. Strauss *et al.* comment that not only does some clinical and nursing work create discomfort for patients, but 'beside all the discomforts inflicted by the personnel while doing diagnostic and therapeutic tasks, patients' discomforts can be heightened by the hospital environment: it can be noisy, poorly ventilated, too hot or too cold, and full of unpleasant odours' (p. 107). 'Comfort care' is an important component of nursing work, for at least in theory nursing is greatly concerned with alleviating the more depersonalized aspects of hospital care. The 'care' component of nursing work may be largely invisible to others, and in consequence is more vulnerable to erosion than other, more visible aspects of nursing work.

Two other types of work which nurses are also heavily involved in are 'sentimental' and 'articulation' work. Articulation work simply refers to the often complex tasks of knitting together and coordinating the variety of tasks and activities which occur in hospital settings. While doctors plan clinical work nurses articulate and coordinate it, and without such work hospital life would come to a halt. Sentimental work extends beyond the alleviation of painful and distressing symptoms and the giving of 'tender loving care' and includes such things as maintaining a patient's trust, orienting the patient to what is happening to them and explaining possible outcomes, helping patients to maintain or recover composure, and, to be discussed more fully below, 'awareness context work', which occurs 'whenever staff withhold information which they believe will be difficult for the ill person to handle' (p. 139). The following chapters are primarily concerned with this type of work and its interrelation with other aspects of nursing.

Another way of looking at the complexity of hospital organization is by a brief specification of the main areas of activity which take place within them (Perrow 1965; Tuckett 1976). As a prerequisite to the clinical work of hospitals, the basic 'hotel functions' of catering, cleaning, laundry, and so on must be provided together with the clinically related services of laboratories, radiology, and the like. Staff must be hired, assigned to units, and paid. Goods and equipment, both 'durables' such as monitoring machines, and 'consumables' such as drugs and syringes, must be ordered, serviced, and delivered to the appropriate work sites. The provision and coordination of this range of goods and services may be quite complicated and difficult to maintain at a satisfactory and predictable level (especially in times of tight financial budgets), yet without them the treatment and care of patients is impossible.

Clinical work is seen as the rationale for hospitals by most people. The clinical treatment of patients with the aim of restoration of normal functioning or maximal rehabilitation, often involving the use of expensive drugs and complicated technology, assumes a central position in hospital life. This area of activity is the main province of medical staff who are supported in their work by nursing staff and a host of other workers. The predominance of chronic disease conditions within modern hospitals makes the goal of complete cure and recovery difficult to achieve in most circumstances, and may make clinical work very complex and difficult to orchestrate (Strauss *et al.* 1985). Although chronic illness predominates, most doctors, it seems, operate with an 'acute care' philosophy, which may mean that incurable and terminally ill patients are seen by them as unrewarding, and so receive less attention from them. Certainly acute services receive proportionally more resources at all levels (not just clinical) than chronic services (DHSS 1983; Garner 1979).

Related to and usually subordinated to clinical therapy is patient care. Indeed the two are only analytically separable in everyday hospital life. Care, which refers to the attention paid to the physiological, psychological, and social needs of patients, is an essential component in the treatment of all patients and is primarily the province of nursing staff. It is especially important and central for the terminally ill, particularly at that point when interventionist aspects of the clinical treatment of disease become subordinated to the requirements of 'palliative care' as such patients near the end of their lives. The 'professionalization' of nursing around the 'care' dimension via the emphasis upon individualized patient care and the introduction of the 'nursing process' has enhanced the importance of patient care as an aspect of hospital work while also increasing the area of potential dispute between doctors and experienced nursing staff over patient management.

Another important area of activity in most British hospitals is the training of new staff. Hospitals are important sites for the training of health care workers, and the presence of large numbers of trainees has a profound effect on patient treatment and management. Indeed, in some settings trainees (house staff, student and pupil nurses) may provide the main source of labour. A number of consequences result from both the reliance of hospitals on staff in training to provide a significant part of their work force and the use of patients as 'learning material' for such staff (Atkinson 1981; Backer *et al.* 1982; Melia 1987; Olesen and Whitaker 1968; Quint 1967). The constant flow of trainees through the wards and units may present some problems of continuity in ward functioning and to a lesser extent patient management as new staff have to 'learn the ropes' of the work setting. Mistakes inevitably occur, which can lead to patient discomfort and even clinical danger. Also, patient selection and choice of treatment may be affected to some extent by training.

A final area to consider is that of research. With the ever increasing specialization of modern medicine and its dependence upon high-level technology, hospitals have become the main sites for the research development of clinical medicine. Not only clinicians but a variety of other researchers can be found in hospitals. As with teaching, the aims and requirements of such research activities are different from and may conflict with the goals of patient treatment and care. As with teaching, research requirements may affect the selection and treatment of patients, and may divert staff and resources from other hospital activities.

These general features of hospitals bear directly and indirectly upon patient treatment and care, and the ways in which patients experience hospitalization. To coordinate these diverse activities requires rules and routines whereby staff work can be coordinated and controlled. For example the collection, collation, and distribution of information about patients – which is central to their treatment and care – cannot be left to chance or purely individual action but requires some systematic control and coordination. The various formal rules and routines provide the framework within which nursing (and other) work takes place, but these are amplified by informal arrangements. Both formal and informal arrangements are continuously negotiated by staff (Strauss *et al.* 1985; Strauss 1978; Strauss *et al.* 1963), and these negotiations are as important as the formal rules and organizational structures themselves – hospitals are not fixed and immutable, but rather are 'structures in process' (Glaser and Strauss 1968). Indeed, given their complexity, continual negotiation and communication between staff both within and between the various work sites of the hospital are essential. Such activities will directly affect the quality of patient care.

THE ORGANIZATION OF HOSPITALS
AND CARE OF THE DYING

Hinton's analysis (1979) of the costs and benefits to the terminally ill of dying at home, in a hospital, or in a hospice clearly demonstrates that different settings may produce differing patterns of cost and benefit for those who are dying. Thus, *where* dying takes place is an important variable. This section looks at hospitals, the next considers hospice care, while the situation of those people dying at home will be discussed briefly in Chapter six.

There are a number of features of hospital life which bear directly on the nursing of dying patients in hospital which are briefly considered here. More extensive discussion can be found in Glaser and Strauss (1965, 1968), Mauksch (1975), McIntosh (1977), and Sudnow (1967), whose work is drawn upon in various ways. Different organizational contexts (wards, units) are characterized by different rhythms and flows of work, and have different (or no) routines for coping with death and dying. They will also vary in the resources available, the number of staff and their training, staff turnover, and management structure, all of which will affect nurse–patient relationships. In general more resources of all kinds are allocated to the 'acute' services (where 75 per cent of all deaths occur), and thus dying patients on 'chronic' services such as geriatrics will have fewer resources, including nursing staff, available for their care.

The care of people who are dying also depends in part on the characteristics of both 'normal' and dying patients on different units. Death on a coronary care unit is very different for staff than death on an acute surgical ward, or on a general medical ward. In the former death is to a certain extent to be expected and staff can psychologically 'offset' such deaths against their many successful recoveries. On the surgical ward, the discovery of a terminal cancer at a routine operation may severely disrupt the 'sentimental order' of the ward, and an unexpected death on the operating table certainly will. On the medical ward death will, as in coronary care, be expected, but the process of dying typically will be more extended and involve older patients than in the other two settings. Glaser and Strauss discuss such differences fully in their work, emphasizing that the period of time over which death occurs and its predictability are major factors affecting how staff treat the dying patient. Another important characteristic is the age of the patient. In our society it is easier for staff to accept the death of elderly patients. In particular, young dying children are psychologically difficult to nurse (Backer *et al.* 1982; Benoliel 1983; Hale *et al.* 1984; Kalish and Reynolds 1977; Quint 1967).

In *Awareness of Dying* (1965) Glaser and Strauss distinguish between 'quick' and 'slow' dying trajectories, and note the different organizational features of such trajectories. Generally deaths which occur over a short span are easier for hospital staff to cope with than slow deaths (but not for the family or friends of the deceased), unless they are unexpected. Quick deaths most commonly occur in emergency and intensive care situations where outcomes quickly become apparent. Most deaths in hospitals are not of this nature, and slow dying is more common and more problematic for doctors and nurses. It is this type of dying trajectory in particular which generates the various problems associated with awareness and disclosure of dying. In slow dying the person is on a lingering downward trajectory, with symptoms often becoming worse and harder to manage. Not only may there be technical aspects of care which are difficult to coordinate and manage, such as balancing various drug regimes, but these also often have a 'moral overlay'. How long, for instance, should life be prolonged by the use of uncomfortable invasive treatment when it is known that recovery is impossible?

One critical dimension to the care of those who are dying is knowledge of the fact and duration of dying: Do staff know? Does the patient know? This is not necessarily straightforward, for the clarity and certainty of both the time and fact of death have become blurred with the predominance of chronic disease and the capacity of modern medicine to intervene in disease processes to avert and retard the dying process (Culver and Gert 1982; Veatch 1976). Sudnow in his discussion of the 'problematic notion' of dying makes a useful distinction between 'clinical death' – the appearance of 'death signs' upon physical examination (e.g. cessation of heart function, flat ECG); 'biological death' – the cessation of cellular activity; and 'social death' – which is 'that point at which socially relevant attributes of the patient begin permanently to cease to be operative as conditions for treating him, and when he is, essentially, regarded as already dead' (1967:74). He provides a number of graphic examples of terminally ill patients being treated as socially dead, for example pre-wrapping and binding of patients' feet for delivery to the morgue. It seems reasonable to suggest that there may be a process of 'social dying' for the terminally ill as others withdraw from social interaction with them, a view supported by Glaser and Strauss's work. What is clear is

25

that certainty of death may develop slowly over a long period of time, that even when the fact of death is certain its timing may remain in doubt, and that 'social death' may often precede 'biological death' (Glaser and Strauss 1965, 1968; Sudnow 1967).

Glaser and Strauss make a persuasive case that the management and disclosure of dying are central to the psycho-social care which dying patients receive. They identify four types of situations or contexts in the management and awareness of dying: closed awareness, suspicion awareness, mutual pretence, and open awareness. Closed awareness refers to the situation where staff (and possibly relatives) know that the patient is terminally ill but the patient does not. The difficulty with this type of awareness context is that of maintaining the context with non-comatose patients, and it is in this type of situation that 'social death' is most likely to occur. Most patients are not sufficiently experienced to recognize the signs of impending death, and their families often concur with or request the withholding of the terminal prognosis from them. Further, as Glaser and Strauss point out,

> hospitals are admirably arranged both by accident and by design, to hide medical information from patients. Records are kept out of reach. Staff are skilled at withholding information. Medical talk about patients generally occurs in far-removed places, and if it occurs nearby, it is couched in medical jargon. Staff members are trained to discuss with patients only the surface aspects of their illness and . . . they are accustomed to acting collusively around patients so as not to disclose medical secrets. The power of the hospital personnel over the patients is vast, since the patients are at their professional mercy for recovery and for such personal everyday requisites as feeding, washing, and even being turned in their beds. (1965:31)

Despite all the above, it seems that most terminally ill patients will eventually move from a closed awareness context to one of the other types of awareness of dying. For example, Hinton (1980) found that 66 per cent of his sample of dying patients indicated to him that they knew they were dying – although they had not necessarily revealed this knowledge to hospital staff or to their relatives.

There are several factors which may lead the dying person to a growing awareness of their impending death. They may become suspicious about their condition due to bodily changes and/or their physical deterioration. In particular certain physical signs, such as lumps or sores which fail to heal, may be believed to be signs of cancer, and hence indicative of possible danger. Changes in treatment regimes are another cue for patients. Changes in behaviour of staff and relatives towards the patient, especially nonverbal signs of stress and general avoidance of talk about 'the future' provide another important set of cues. In the study by Knight and Field (1981) which is summarized in Chapter three it was found that the most important cues for dying patients related to their clinical treatment and to the lack of clear diagnosis.

Closed awareness most frequently breaks down into suspicion, which may be very destructive for staff–patient and patient–relative relationships. It is in this awareness context that patients may engage in a variety of behaviours aimed at 'trapping' staff and relatives into revealing that their suspicions are correct. Patients in this state may also be very alert to various cues which indicate that all is not well. There may be a mutual pretence in which all parties 'deny' the fact of impending death, and references to the future may be dropped and talk restricted to 'safe topics'. This may solve the interactional problems of closed awareness and suspicion. It may not, however, allow what Kubler-Ross (1970, 1975) refers to as the final 'stage' of dying – acceptance of one's own death – since the patient will be unable to discuss it with others. Of course, it is possible that different types of awareness will exist between a patient and the various people with whom s/he is in contact, as Hinton's research confirms (Hinton 1980).

In the introduction it was suggested that there appears to be a move towards open awareness as the preferred type of relationship between patients who are dying and hospital staff. In an open context the fact of death is known by all parties, and as far as possible so is the likely time of death. In this context patients may become involved in decisions about the management of their care (although not all will choose to do so), and can make practical arrangements for their impending death (e.g. making a will, settling business affairs). One of the problems this book addresses is which features of nursing work best facilitate an open awareness context? It should be emphasized that although open awareness is now seen by many caregivers to be the most desirable situation, all situations pose difficulties for nurses. While open awareness reduces some of the problems stemming from avoidance, evasion, suspicion, and pretence, other problems regarding, for example, discussions of when death might occur or planning for the patient's remaining future may well occur (Bond and Bond 1986:262–6).

One of the Glaser and Strauss team, Quint (1967), in *The Nurse and the Dying Patient*, focused upon student nurses. She was highly critical of the training nurses receive to deal with their encounters with dying patients, noting that 'there were few teachers who offered guidance in how to talk to dying patients' (p. 40). Teaching staff were inexperienced in and uncomfortable about nursing dying people, while on the wards students learnt from experienced nurses to minimize their personal involvement with dying patients and their relatives. Conversations with dying patients were difficult because of lack of direction from teachers and more experienced nurses. In particular conversations when patients were suspicious or wanted to talk openly about their dying were difficult for nurses. Prolonged contact and personal identification and involvement with dying patients were also sources of difficulty for nurses. Because nurses found it hard, received no support or encouragement to talk with patients who were dying, and had to rely on their own resources, they learnt to limit the time they spent with dying patients, to avoid them, and to restrict their involvement with them. Given all this it is unsurprising that 'many nurses get little personal satisfaction from the interactions with dying patients' (Quint 1967:196).

Two British studies suggest that it is possible to generalize the findings of the Glaser and Strauss team to the British situation. McIntosh's study (1977) drew upon their work and focused on the management of information about cancer. The practice of the doctors on the ward studied was to avoid disclosure to all patients, and various strategies to keep diagnosis from them, such as the use of euphemistic terms, were developed. The nurses were kept informed of diagnosis and treatment and shared and endorsed this policy of avoidance. Even if they felt that a patient should be informed that they had cancer they did not consider it their place to do so. More recently Bond (1982, 1983) studied nurses' communication with cancer patients. Again doctors believed that disclosure of the diagnosis of cancer or of prognosis should be avoided and, as in the McIntosh study, a number of ambiguous expressions and routine explanations were developed to allow them to avoid such disclosure. Direct information about patients was not communicated to the nurses, but they assumed that patients had not been informed of their diagnosis or prognosis. 'In the main they shared the doctors' beliefs about the harmfulness of disclosure because of cancer patients' pessimistic conceptions' (Bond 1983:68). Bond reports that personal problems or social matters were rarely discussed with patients, and that nurses did not see this as part of their role. Nursing work was task oriented, with all nurses sharing responsibility for all patients, and most nurse–patient interactions were primarily concerned with physical care and treatment. Such nursing practices 'which sought to avoid reference to cancer or its implications, were not helpful to patients who attempted to acquire information or establish mutuality about their feelings [although] they did succeed in perpetuating denial and uncertainty among those utilizing this coping strategy' (Bond 1983:71).

HOSPICE CARE

The modern hospice movement for the care of dying people began largely as a reaction against the depersonalized care of dying people in hospitals. It can arbitrarily be said to have started with the founding of St Christopher's Hospice by Cicely Saunders in 1967, although hospice care of the dying has existed for centuries. The hospices emphasized a completely different set of priorities in their care of dying people to those found in hospitals. The aim was to provide person-centred 'holistic' care of dying patients' social, physical, psychological, and spiritual needs. Unlike hospitals hospices accepted emotional involvement as a natural and important part of the relationship between caregivers and those who were dying, and provided support systems to enable their staff to cope with such involvement. Because emotion and sentiment were important ingredients of hospice care, carers were not restricted to those who had technical skills and training. Initially hospices aimed to involve everyone in the care of dying people in a nonhierarchical team of carers which included medical professionals, nurses, clergy, volunteers, and the patients' relatives. Patients were to be fully involved in decisions about their care, the emphasis of which was on the quality of life. Consequently care was to be geared towards palliative treatment of symptoms with the aim of making 'the life that remains' free from distress. The hospice itself was to provide peaceful and homelike surroundings, with unrestricted visiting and a minimum of formal rules and arrangements (Saunders *et al.* 1981; Twycross 1986).

The early hospices were primarily in-patient institutions, but there is now a wide range of hospice services, encompassing day centres, in-hospital support teams, and out-patient and home support services. Since the mid-1970s the hospice idea has become very popular, with a dramatic growth in in-patient and support teams since 1975 (Seale 1989). Hospice ideals have also had an impact in North America, which has witnessed a similar increase in a great variety of hospice programmes over the same time scale (Abel 1986), and in Australia, Europe, and New Zealand. The hospices appear to have been very successful in achieving their ideals, and to have owed their success primarily to their dedicated and proficient staff. In terms of symptom management one of the outstanding achievements of the movement has been its contribution to pain control in the terminally ill. They have demonstrated the close interconnection between physical and psychological distress, showing that anxiety and depression can be markedly reduced by good control of pain and other symptoms (Twycross 1978). They have also shown that it is possible to talk with people who are dying and their relatives about death without adverse consequences. Indeed the hospices are strong proponents of the beneficial consequences of such openness. These successes of the hospices appear to have influenced the care of people dying in our hospitals in only unsystematic and partial ways.

Despite their successes concerns are being expressed that the initial ideals and high standards are no longer being sustained in some hospice organizations (Abel 1986; James 1986; Seale 1989). In-patient hospice care is an expensive and labour-intensive form of care and financial constraints are one element which has led to the diversity of organizational forms which hospices now take, especially in the United States. Where costs are shared by health authorities or, in the United States, by other health providers, their demands and expectations may constrain work practices in ways which compromise the initial hospice ideals. Hospices are dependent upon their staff for delivering the high-quality, person-centred care which their ethos demands, yet where staff are shared with the rest of the hospital it may be impossible to guarantee that they will share the important underlying philosophy of care. James (1986) suggests that the shift of emphasis from holistic care towards physical care in the hospice which she studied was partly the result of its loss of 'specialness' as it became integrated with its host NHS hospital. Hospices may no longer provide as high a level of support for their staff as earlier, with consequent problems for managing staff stress and 'burnout'. Finally, the hospices are vulnerable to the processes and institutionalization and rationalization once the dedicated and 'charismatic' idealists who were responsible for their foundation and the first cadre of highly selected staff leave (Weber 1947; Abel 1986; James 1986). Concerns such as these have led to calls for evaluation of hospices and their organizational functioning (Seale 1989).

While the hospices have served as 'demonstration models' of good terminal care, and have been responsible for the training of many caregivers in terminal care, they cannot provide the main source of care for dying people and will not replace homes and hospitals as the places where most dying people will be cared for, at least in the forseeable future. Hospices depend on high staff–patient ratios, and despite the extensive use of volunteers require comparatively large numbers of well-trained and highly motivated nurses. They are thus expensive. Apart from being expensive forms of care, hospices quite simply cannot meet the total demand. They have been primarily concerned with the care of those dying from cancer, and seem reluctant to admit other types of dying patients in large numbers, for example people dying from AIDS. Rather than create more in-patient hospices in Britain the Wilkes review (1980) recommended better provision of domicilary services and liaison with other services. The incorporation of hospice ideals and methods into hospital care of those who are dying, especially with reference to symptom management, communication with patients, and support of caregivers, also seems highly desirable.

SUMMARY

The main purpose of the first two chapters has been to introduce some orienting ideas and to review relevant background material in preparation for the remainder of the book. The nursing care which people dying in our hospitals receive is not simply the product of decisions and actions of individual nurses. At the most general level nurses are influenced in the ways in which they relate to dying people by the fearful and apprehensive attitudes towards death and dying which seem to be widespread in our society. Their actions are also likely to be influenced by the training which they receive and the way in which the occupation of nursing is organized. The care of dying patients is directly influenced by methods of organizing and allocating nursing work within hospitals. This in turn is affected by the complexity of the organization of modern hospitals, which leads to the development of routines whereby staff can organize their work in a predictable manner and cope with the demands placed upon them. The general and specific working relationships between nurses and doctors are particularly influential in the development of work routines. Unfortunately the personal needs of patients may be overlooked in the pursuit of these routines. A particular goal of these chapters was to consider the problems surrounding the disclosure of a terminal condition to a dying person. This is clearly not something which nurses find easy, but the awareness of patients about whether they are dying, and the nature of communication with their caregivers is seen to be of central importance to the quality of their care. These matters will be discussed in greater detail in Chapter seven after we have presented the details of our research.

Part Two

NURSING THE DYING

We had a patient who was here over a year – and we were
all very close to 'C'. I saw him from when he came in, to
getting really better, then going down again . . . It was
awful because there was nothing I could do – I just had to
sit and hold his hand. At that time we were all taking it in
turns to sit with him as long as we could 'cos we just didn't
want him to die on his own. Nobody wanted just to go in
and find him dead. Which I think goes for most of the
patients that you know are on their last legs. You don't
want to leave them on their own. . . . I remember very
clearly a patient on geriatrics. I had nursed him on nights,
and I went back on to days – he was a double-sided CVA.
He was very incoherent. By some miracle he could just
whisper words. And at night he couldn't sleep because he
was so uncomfortable so I used to spend a lot of my nights
sitting and talking to him and holding his hand. When I
went back on to days I went behind the curtains – and he
was really on his last legs. So I just sat with him and held
his hand. And I remember the staff nurse coming in and
asking me if I had nothing better to do. So I said, 'No. Not
at this moment, no.' So she said, 'Would you mind going
and finding something to do?' I remember it so clearly. I
really hated her; because this man was dying. I'd been with
him all this time, and why should he die alone? All she was
content with was giving him BPO's and he still had an
enema the day he did die. Well he died that afternoon. I felt
awful – this poor little man – and just as I went behind the
curtains he just said – he grabbed hold of my arms (he got

33

very little movement in that hand), and he just put his hand on mine and whispered, 'I love you.' And then he died in the afternoon. I thought, 'Well, it's all worthwhile', because at least he realized that somebody cared.

RE, Staff Nurse on Ward 6

'A silent conspiracy': nursing terminally ill cancer patients on an acute surgical ward

The purpose of this chapter is to open the discussion of problems associated with nursing dying patients by briefly presenting what might be termed a 'typical' example of such work. It introduces the two central themes of the study: the problems surrounding dying patients' awareness of dying, and how the organization of nursing work affects their interaction and communication with nurses. The chapter reports on a participant-observation study of an acute surgical ward at Midland General Hospital. The data was collected by Mary Knight (MK), who worked as a nursing auxiliary on the ward during the summer of 1979 and whom the author supervised. Using this method meant that it was not necessary to disclose that the study was being undertaken, and therefore communication and general behaviour were natural and normal. MK was able to experience at first hand the inherent difficulties of nursing dying patients, and to analyse colleagues' attitudes towards the terminally ill. Furthermore, since we had access to the patient's notes we were aware of their diagnosis and prognosis. The limitations of such a method were that only a limited view of ward functioning could be obtained, and that a systematic examination of nurses' attitudes was precluded. The chapter serves as a contrast to the findings presented in subsequent chapters and illustrates what may be termed the 'traditional' way of coping with the terminally ill in hospitals.

This chapter is based on Knight and Field (1981).

THE WARD

Ward 7 was a typical surgical ward containing 27 beds catering for male and female patients. It was a 'harness style' ward comprising five bays each containing four or six beds and some individual rooms. Sexes were not mixed in four bays although the fifth 'acute bay' on occasions contained both sexes, who were often heavily sedated or comatose. Patient turnover was high (in one week 64 patients spent time on the ward), and this rapid turnover was a major factor contributing to a strict adherence to routine by the nursing staff in order to cope with the numerous daily admissions, the three days a week which were the theatre days, the days when the ward was accepting emergency admissions, and the day-to-day nursing needs of the ever changing patient population. Doctor-nurse relationships were very formal and hierarchical, with consultants and other surgical staff talking only to the sister or charge nurse. This was mirrored by a similarly formal ranking of nursing staff.

The ward was short of fully trained nursing staff. Many of them were undergoing their training, and of the regular staff three were nursing auxiliaries. Thus unqualified and trainee nurses made up the majority of nurses on the ward. The work was generally undertaken by these junior nurses on a 'task allocation' basis, that is nurses were given tasks such as taking temperatures or giving bed baths which covered the whole ward, rather than being allocated to look after all the needs of a few patients. The Sister or most senior staff nurse conducted the ward administration in her office. Ward 7 was not a terminal ward, and so there was little thought by the patients that they might die, and among the staff there were problems of acceptance when a patient returned from surgery where a fatal malignancy had been discovered. Nurses were forbidden by the surgeons to disclose a terminal prognosis to a patient even if asked.

THE PATIENT SAMPLE

From the 40 terminally ill patients admitted to the ward during the study period the 13 with whom MK had greatest contact during her work were studied intensively. This group comprised eight males and five females whose cancer had been considered inoperable and terminal by the surgeons. Six of these patients died on the ward and the other seven were either sent home or to a place of residential care to die. Twelve of the patients were admitted without a doctor's awareness that they had cancer and without being themselves aware of this. The majority arrived optimistic that their condition would be investigated and rectified, and after a period of time these patients, both those who had had surgery and those who had not, began to question why they were not getting better and in some cases why they were deteriorating daily. One patient was aware of her illness and its terminal implications for her cancer had been detected 18 months earlier, and she had returned to hospital because her family could not cope with her care at home.

RECOGNIZING IMPENDING DEATH

Twenty per cent of all patients entering Ward 7 were admitted for investigation without a diagnosis having been made, and the majority of patients who later proved to have terminal cancer came from this group. A small proportion of cancer patients were out-patients whose condition had been misdiagnosed, and who were found to have cancer after tests or during surgery. An important feature of any diagnosis, whether correctly established or not, is that it involves questions of definition. Anyone may read the medical signs and draw their own conclusions, the terminal patient included. However, in British hospitals the attending doctor is the only one who can legitimately define the patient's condition, and ordinarily only s/he may tell patients that they are dying. Nevertheless, the nurses on Ward 7 had to assess whether a patient was dying and when s/he was likely to die, and making such assessments was often no easy matter. In reaching their conclusion nurses might make their own interpretation of cues – how the patient looked and acted, what the charts reported – as well as relying on information and cues given, perhaps unwittingly and obliquely, by surgeons. Typically they tended to trust this latter source more than their own individual or collective interpretation. The particularly poor communication between surgical and nursing staff on Ward 7 heightened the relevance for nurses of their own observations and thus, although the most legitimate source of expectations about death were the surgeons, the nurses also observed their own cues constantly (Glaser and Strauss (1965) give a good account of this type of activity).

Nurses' definitions of patients' illness status affected their behaviour towards them, and so the time when these definitions changed was significant. Glaser and Strauss (1968) discuss this period when a cancer is discovered in terms of a decrease in alertness by nurses. This was to some extent true of Ward 7, but the greater change in behaviour towards the dying patient concerned the personal attention the patient received. In the majority of cases observed this increased considerably. In one case after a patient returned from surgery where a malignancy had been discovered the nurses' attitudes towards her changed so dramatically that she became suspicious of her diagnosis. Prior to her operation she had received minimal attention since most nurses felt she exaggerated her symptoms; after the operation nurses increased their attention to her, apparently to compensate for their feelings of guilt about their previous attitudes.

The most obvious influence on patients' awareness about their terminal condition is the doctors' policy of informing the patient about the nature of his or her condition. Where the practice is to inform patients they are likely to manifest an 'open awareness' perspective, where they are not told – as on Ward 7 – a greater proportion of them will possess a 'closed awareness' or 'suspicion awareness' perspective. In every case observed, not merely those patients in the sample, the surgical staff on Ward 7 did not inform the patients that they had cancer, although they always informed the relatives of the terminal prognosis. However, there was occasionally a breakdown in communication between relatives and surgical staff because of the use of euphemisms which the staff presumed relatives would take to mean 'cancer'. Surgeons frequently felt that they had enlightened relatives when in fact they were no better informed than before. Families typically did not tell patients that they were dying, nor did they wish them to be told by hospital staff (a commonly reported phenomenon).

On Ward 7 none of the patients observed (including those outside the core group of 13) had any allies who revealed to them or helped them to discover their impending death. Not only staff and families, but other patients on the ward who knew or guessed that a patient was dying colluded in the withholding of information. It seemed that when patients wanted less distressing information or support they could readily find allies among the other patients; when they were dying the others followed normal rules of tact, keeping their knowledge to themselves or at least away from the dying patients. Thus, the situation of these patients could be aptly described as one where they existed within a conspiracy of silence. Yet despite this 'closed awareness' context only five of the 13 core patients seemed to be completely unaware of their condition.

There were numerous cues, as Glaser and Strauss (1965) and McIntosh (1977) have pointed out, which could lead patients to become suspicious that their condition was not what it was purported to be, and which could lead them to suspect they had cancer. They might be alerted by their symptoms, or compare their condition with that of a relative or friend who had had cancer. A swift admission associated with 'cancer treatment', particularly referral for radiotherapy, was another important cue. Finally, their own physical deterioration was an important cue that something was seriously wrong. In addition to these patient-centered cues there were verbal and behavioural cues from staff which they could observe and attempt to elicit. Following Kelly and Friesen (1950) three main strategies of information-seeking were identified. First, patients could pay special attention to the conversation around them, especially during ward rounds. Next, they could directly query staff, and although this would not lead directly to answers could uncover validating clues. Third, they could use indirect questions to 'set traps' for the staff. If the staff were successfully to maintain dying patients in a state of ignorance they had to remain on guard against accidentally revealing by their speech or behaviour that all was not well. Such cues were particularly likely to be disclosed when staff were unaware that patients were suspicious about their condition. Thus it was essential that staff fully discussed among themselves patients' conditions, and whether they were showing signs of suspicion. However, as communication between different levels of staff was poor this did not occur, and the lack of such communication increased the likelihood of patients learning about their terminal prognosis by mistake. While staff persisted in presenting a hopeful picture to the patient, even to the extent of continuing 'restorative' treatment, inconsistencies and verbal slips often undermined this picture.

The most important cues from surgical staff related to treatment and lack of clear diagnosis. Where the surgeon did not give an explicit recognizable label to the condition when the patient had assumed an unthreatening diagnosis, the patient would interpret this as something more sinister. Some forms of treatment were known by some patients to be associated with cancer, and this served as an important source of cues. Not only the type of treatment, but also the time taken to reach a decision regarding the appropriate form of treatment and the type of operation were also cues. A second operation often led a patient to adopt a gloomy outlook. In the same vein, supplementary treatment was considered a bad sign. Tests undergone after an operation were also feared. Clues from nurses came primarily from inconsistencies in their accounts to patients and from sudden changes in their attitudes towards them. Junior nurses in particular were likely to reveal such inconsistencies and to be 'trapped' by patients into doing so.

RELATIONSHIPS ON THE WARD

The relationships on the ward, not only between hospital personnel and patients, but also between surgical and nursing staff, played a significant part in the awareness of patients and the ways in which nurses related to them. The strict adherence to routine and the system of task allocation of nursing work had two main consequences. It made it hard for the nursing staff to become familiar with the up to 27 patients on the ward, and for long-stay patients, obviously including the terminally ill patients, it created problems of disorientation. Their 'friends' in the beds near by were forever changing and, since the ward was divided into bays of patients of the same sex, they were themselves moved from one bay to another.

There was a clear division of nursing labour on the ward. The qualified senior nurses took little direct part in patient care and were mainly occupied with administration and management of the ward. Third-year student nurses were mainly concerned with the treatment of acute care patients who were often undergoing very sophisticated treatment. The care of those who were dying fell to junior nurses largely as a result of this division of labour. These nurses were not allowed into Sister's office for refuge from working pressures, which reinforced their estrangement from the other nurses, and was an element in the close relationships they tended to develop with long-stay patients. The Sister was seen as a 'battle-axe' by both patients and junior nurses and they received sympathy from each other after unpleasant encounters with her. This bond meant that where patients were anxious about their condition they were more likely to question these nurses, whom they considered to be their friends, than other staff.

The surgical staff on Ward 7 had very little communication with any of the nurses except the Sister, and maintained an aloofness which was unhelpful to junior nurses in situations where they felt that a senior doctor ought to know about a patient's anxieties. This meant that some information of this kind was not related to surgical staff. Rounds on Ward 7 were conducted by a consultant and the ward Sister or her deputy. He would go to all the beds in the ward, including those of his colleague where he typically spent less time than with his own patients. It was evident that he spent more time at beds where patients had been operated upon recently. It was also evident that where surgery had been unsuccessful surgical staff spent less time with patients (Roth (1963) reported similar behaviour in his study of TB hospitals). Once patients with inoperable cancer returned to the ward from theatre, and their drugs had been prescribed, doctors rarely asked any more than 'Are you in pain?'. The question of going home was avoided, as was any discussion with the patient about the operation. In the climate of Ward 7, which was geared to repair and recovery, the dying cancer patient was a medical 'failure'. Such patients became anxious when their conversation with the consultant was brief, and invariably once the surgeons had left the ward they would question the nursing staff about their condition, asking why the doctors had shown less interest in them than in other patients.

The care of dying patients fell largely by default to first-year student nurses, pupil nurses, and the nursing auxiliaries. These nurses had the greatest contact with, and greatest trust placed in them by, the patients. It was not uncommon for these nurses to form close bonds with the (long-stay) terminally ill patients, even with the 'awkward characters' because they spent so much time with them, and several patients looked on the junior nurses as confidants. This was mainly due to patients' awareness that their fellow patients might have grave problems related to their illness. They therefore preferred to discuss their own illness with nurses whom they presumed to have knowledge and understanding of it, and even of their psycho-social problems. These relationships were often experienced as very demanding by the young trainee nurses, many of whom would not have resolved their own attitudes towards death and dying (cf. Charles-Edwards 1983; Simpson 1975). Although there were many factors involved in concealing their condition from dying patients, there were also pressures upon the junior nurses as a result of their close relationships and frequent contact with dying patients to be truthful with them. This was especially difficult to cope with when a patient was overtly anxious and in need of reassurance.

COMMUNICATION ON THE WARD

The general principle underlying staff–patient interactions was that staff were superior by virtue of their greater knowledge and status. Once this was established, usually unproblematically, communication between staff and patient became routinized and mainly restricted to 'technical' matters. In this sense it was very similar to the communication patterns reported by Bond (1982, 1983) and McIntosh (1977). Such routinization contributed to the management of communication in three main ways. First, it ensured consistency in the sort of communication which a patient or patients with similar conditions received from any staff member. Second, surgeons were absolved from having to take decisions on individual cases – their responses to questions appeared to be generally routinized irrespective of the character of the patient. Third, it ensured that members of staff did not come into conflict over what patients should be told. In particular it was understood by all staff that patients should not be given unfavourable information about their condition. However, despite all this there were sometimes severe problems in interaction with the dying cancer patients, especially for junior nurses who were often explicitly asked by them if they had cancer.

The pressures of working with dying patients were very demanding not only in terms of the amount of nursing care required but also because the nurses felt that they could not allow themselves to become over-involved with any one patient. Further, they received no formal education about the psychological needs of the dying person or how to come to terms with impending death (the local nursing school has subsequently provided some instruction in its basic courses). As Quint (1967) points out, although young nurses are taught how to care for patients physically and sometimes 'psychologically' they are rarely taught how to cope with conversations about death and dying.

The problems of coping with and accepting imminent death provided two basic problems for the junior nursing staff on Ward 7. First, it was very difficult for them to talk frankly about death with the dying person. No matter how many similar situations they may have witnessed it was hard for them to reassure the dying person when they had not come to terms with their own death. Most nurses had not thought of their own death seriously, and for some of them nursing people who were dying raised questions which remained largely unresolved. Simpson (1975) reported similar findings, and DF also found this to be the case with some of the younger nurses whom he interviewed. This problem occurred even with the patient who was fully aware of and resigned to her impending death. The problem was accentuated by the insistence of surgical staff upon maintaining a closed awareness context, for in this situation nurses had to come to terms with reassuring patients, who were confused and anxious about their physical deterioration, that they would recover when they knew that in fact they would not do so. This was distressing for the young nurses, especially when they had built up a relationship with the patient. There were two common strategies whereby junior nurses could evade patients' question while maintaining a friendly relationship with them. The organization of work on the ward in terms of tasks made it possible for them to be working elsewhere and thus physically to avoid contact with the patient and/or suggest that they were too busy to talk. Secondly, they could legitimately plead ignorance of the patient's case by virtue of their low status in the ward hierarchy and refer the patient to a more senior nurse or to a doctor. In their studies Sudnow (1967) and Quint (1967) found this latter strategy was the most common way of dealing with questions from dying patients. Communication patterns on the ward reinforced and supported such evasion.

A major factor inhibiting communication between dying patients and surgical staff was the great respect and deference shown them by patients, a phenomenon reported by Cartwright (1967) in her general survey of hospital care. Junior nursing staff often suggested to patients who expressed confusion about their condition they they should 'ask the consultant about it', but patients were afraid to do so because 'He's a very busy man'. One woman said that he (the consultant) would think her stupid if she asked him to explain her condition to her because he had already done so and she had not understood him. In fact the consultant had not explained her condition (terminal cancer) to her but had evaded the issue by talking about 'complications' thus confusing her more. These barriers were harmful from the surgeon's point of view: patients usually dressed up and cheered up for the consultants but rarely discussed their anxieties with them. These were more often relayed to junior nurses, who had little communication with surgical staff. These nurses felt that they could not tell surgical staff of patient anxieties, because it was hard for the surgeons to accept that a patient who was courteous and relaxed in their presence was to nurses a deeply depressed and anxious character.

These problems tended to alienate further the junior nursing staff from the surgical staff. Although after a period of time nurses knew whether a patient had cancer because of their access to the patient's notes and their recognition of certain forms of treatment, they did not know how much the patient had been told about his or her condition. Thus when patients said, 'I know I've got cancer', the nurse could not be certain that the patient was 'trying her out' and waiting for her reaction, or whether they genuinely knew because they had been told by relatives. In such situations evasion and avoidance of patients were tempting solutions to the nurse's difficulties.

SUMMARY

The main purpose of this chapter has been to introduce some of the themes which run throughout the rest of this work. The central theme concerns the problems surrounding patients' awareness of dying, disclosure of terminality, and communication of nurses with patients. A closely related theme is the organization of nursing work which affects such disclosure, awareness, and communication. The example of Ward 7 shows that withholding the disclosure of terminal prognosis from patients does not guarantee that they will not become aware or suspect that they are dying, a finding which has been well documented (Glaser and Strauss 1965;

Quint 1967; Hinton 1980) and is well known. It is also clear that such a policy creates problems for interaction between nurses and the terminally ill. While pressures may be alleviated for doctors by the withholding of unpleasant information from patients, to a large extent these pressures are merely transferred to nursing staff. In the case of Ward 7 this resulted in poor communications between surgical staff, senior nurses, and junior nurses, with the latter bearing the brunt of such dissimulation. These problems were largely the product of the organization of work on the ward.

Chapter Four

'We didn't want him to die on his own': nursing dying patients on a general medical ward

This chapter is based on interviews with all 16 of the qualified and training nursing staff working days on a 28-bed general medical ward at Midland General. The interviews took place over a seven-week period during May–June 1982 in the vacant night Sister's Office which was located away from the main work areas of the ward. This greatly reduced the opportunity for observation of general nursing work, although some observation was possible, and DF met and talked with a few patients as well as socializing with nurses before and after the interviewing. It was thus possible to gain some partial and nonsystematic evaluation of how nurses' verbal accounts compared with their 'coffee time' talk and their relations with patients.

THE WARD

Ward 6 was a 'harness style' ward with female and male patients segregated by sex in the four- or six-bed bays. During the second week of the study period the mean age of the 33 patients who spent time on the ward was 57; the youngest patient was 19 and the oldest patient 96. Twenty-seven per cent of the patients were under the age of 50 and 42 per cent over the age of 65. During 1982 there were 63 deaths on the ward, but none during the study period. At the time of the study bed occupancy was running at nearly 90 per cent, and was 87.9 per cent for the year. (All information is taken from the Medical Unit report for 1982.) Despite the high level of bed occupancy the rhythm of work on the ward

This chapter is taken from and expands upon Field (1984).

appeared to be generally relaxed, and the attitude that nursing work meant doing something to patients (Clarke 1978) was noticeably absent. During slack times (when most of DF's visits occurred) nurses could typically be found chatting to patients.

Ward 6 was run along team lines, with authority delegated widely among the trained nursing staff. Charge nurse duty rotated among all qualified staff rather than being based simply on seniority (a SEN was in charge at the time of DF's first visit even though two SRNs were also on duty). Trainee nurses were fully involved with patient care and were not relegated to the status of simply an extra pair of hands to perform routine tasks. The delegative and 'permissive' leadership style of the Sister was very evident, and her role appeared to be in large part devoted to supporting the rest of the nursing team (and trying to develop their skills), facilitating their interpersonal relationships with patients where necessary, and mediating between nurses, patients, and doctors. Her leadership style and strongly expressed attitudes were central to the ethos of patient care enacted on the ward.

Nursing work was organized through a system whereby patients were allocated to teams of nurses responsible for all the patients within their bays, and within these teams to individual nurses. The nursing process had been introduced three years previously and was reported by nurses to be working smoothly after some initial problems (McKeown 1980). It was now accepted by all nurses, taken seriously, and believed to be a relevant and useful way of organizing nursing work. The operation of this pattern of work and belief was to make nurses individually responsible for their patients within the context of team and ward support.

> RL I tend to rely on Sister – I go to her and she advises. When it gets sticky we tend to refer to her and then she helps. She sort of goes over the sticky bit then she refers it back to us, because she's very good at that.
> DF And do you do the same for junior nurses?
> RL Oh yes. If they come to us and we feel we can cope with it, we'll cope with it. If we can't we refer it to Sister – we don't try to get out of our depth in it.

Doctor–nurse relationships on Ward 6 were not overly formal and nurses were allowed a good deal of autonomy in their work. Cases were discussed between medical and nursing staff, and the nurses reported that a good relationship existed between them. Medical staff had less active involvement in the care of dying patients than nursing staff, and might withdraw almost entirely once the transition from 'therapeutic cure' to 'relief care' (Saunders 1978) had been decided upon.

In sharp contrast to the research reported in the previous chapter medical staff were willing to accede to nurses' views about the desirability of 'disclosure' of terminal prognosis to patients. For example, a case was recounted by the Sister where medical staff felt that a patient should not be informed that she was terminally ill whereas the nursing staff felt that she should be told. It was agreed that the Sister would tell the patient who, when told, thanked the Sister and made arrangements to ensure that a planned holiday occurred while she was well enough to go. Further, a policy of 'open disclosure' existed on the ward which meant that nurses could inform patients about their diagnosis and prognosis – including that of terminality – without first having to seek permission to do so from the relevant consultant should the occasion arise. The nursing staff were encouraged by the Sister and the Nursing Officer to follow the open disclosure policy. Both the Nursing Officer and the Sister told DF that they regarded helping the nurses in this area as an important part of their roles.

ASPECTS OF DYING

Table 4.1 shows the main topics covered in the interviews and gives a rough indication of the nurses' responses. The similarity of these nurses' attitudes to those reported elsewhere suggest that they were not unusual in their views, and that we can therefore take seriously the findings reported in the next two sections of this chapter. As would be expected they found it easier to accept the death of elderly people than the death of children or young people. All of the trainees and four of the qualified nurses expressed such sentiments. Young deaths were seen as 'wasteful' and in addition many of the nurses presumed that old people 'had had a good life'.

PJ   I think it's more difficult to nurse a younger person than it is to nurse an older person.

DF   Why?

Table 4.1 Nurses' responses to various topics related to nursing dying patients

Aspect	Unqualified (n = 11)	Qualified (n = 7)
Self		
Scared or disturbed by thought of own death	6	0
Had someone close to them die	6	5
Aspects of dying		
Harder to nurse young dying patients	10	4
Elderly assumed to have had 'good life'	7	4
Death sometimes a blessing	8	4
Unexpected death harder to cope with	6	4
Short duration of dying easier to cope with	1	0
No difference between dying and other patients*	1	4
Awareness preferences		
Open	6	6
Closed	1	1
Emotional involvement		
Involved with dying patients	9	7
Problems with involvement	4	0
Involvement unavoidable	5	7
Kept in touch with relatives*	1	4
Ward seen as 'family' for long-term dying patients*	1	6

* Not all nurses referred to these aspects.

PJ Because life is so short for the younger person. With the older person, they've had their time and you can't prolong life for too long. For a younger person it's quite sad.

The qualified nurses were slightly more complex in their reasoning than the trainees. For them it was not merely that the elderly had 'had a good life', but also that they were perceived as more accepting and ready to die.

EW (. . .) I feel you can help an elderly person more than you can a teenager – an elderly person is more *ready* to die, I think. Or accepts it more easily. So they are quite – not happy – but they're ready to take all the comfort you can give them. Whereas a teenager, they're frightened if he thinks, or overhears, or feels that he is going to die. He's very, very, frightened.

Nurses sometimes linked the death of elderly people with the view that death could be a 'blessing' or 'release' for patients, but this was by no means seen as an inevitable link. Death was seen as a release for patients who were suffering from painful or distressing symptoms, often over a long period of time, no matter what their age.

> *SA* (. . .) they kept giving her more blood and she kept throwing it back – she had a lovely personality, she was so caring (. . .) I think the staff felt so sorry for her and felt they wanted her to die because she was having to put up with all this; they didn't want her dead but they wanted her to die so she wouldn't have to suffer.

In their study Glaser and Strauss (1968) found that it was easier for staff to cope with patients who died quickly and expectedly than those who died over a long period of time. Eight nurses said that they found, or anticipated finding, unexpected deaths harder to cope with than expected deaths. However, only one (trainee) nurse indicated that 'quick death' was easier to cope with. The remainder either said that there was no difference or could not indicate how they thought the duration of the 'dying trajectory' would affect their nursing. Some implied that too rapid a death would in fact be harder to cope with as they would not have had a chance to establish a relationship with the person or to provide the patient with 'good nursing care'.

AWARENESS CONTEXTS

As already indicated, a central concern of this study is to examine nurses' views of various 'awareness contexts' (Glaser and Strauss 1965). We have seen in the previous chapter that even in a ward which did not allow the disclosure of terminal prognosis to patients, and where conditions favoured the maintenance of 'closed awareness', patients became aware or suspected that they were dying (Knight and Field 1981). On Ward 6 nurses were not asked directly whether they thought that terminally ill patients knew that they were dying, but eleven of them volunteered views on this during the course of the interview. Nine of them were certain that most dying patients knew that they were dying without directly being told.

RP I think it's easier if they do know to a certain extent. I think even if they haven't been told towards the end they know deep down inside them, and they usually end up telling me they are going to die, then I don't have to tell them.

DF Has that happened to you? Several times, many times?

RP Yes. It's quite common, or it seems to be.

The nurses often adduced examples from their own or other nurses' experiences to support the view that patients 'knew' of their impending death.

PJ I think every dying person has got some sort of insight because you come across some uncanny things (. . .) [like] a patient dying while all the relatives are at home, and the family had just been on holiday and the son had come back from work abroad, and they were all at home (. . .) and he died that day [when] they were all back together as a family.

Contrary to the findings of McIntosh (1977) and the widely held view that a situation of 'closed awareness' is preferred by hospital staff, only two of the nurses said that they thought it was easier to nurse dying patients who were unaware of their impending death. As in the work of Glaser and Strauss (1965, 1968) the majority of nurses who expressed a preference chose 'open awareness'.

SG I think with patients who are dying you have to make a specific judgement on each person whether you think they can handle the information, and also take into consideration the relatives' wishes. But, as a general rule, I'd say yes, if a person asks you and you think they are up to it, to tell. I find it easier then to carry on a relationship with a patient to its termination, rather than having this superficial relationship that suddenly one day he's going – boomp – you're left hanging up in the air.

For the younger trainee nurses such a view was largely anticipatory and they were tentative in their choice. Even for trained staff the preference for 'openness' was not unproblematic, as this staff nurse indicates:

DF So you have no difficulty talking to them?

RL Oh no. Sometimes I find it very difficult if they don't know they're dying, and the relatives have expressed a wish that they're not to be told and the doctors haven't told them yet. You know (. . .) the time when they first get to know. I find that a bit difficult still. It's all right when they don't know. It's the in-between bit when they are getting to know and they're asking some difficult questions.

As this shows, *getting* to the situation of open awareness may be hard, especially for the trainee nurse. It was in this phase of their relationship that the qualified staff saw the ward Sister as playing an important role as a broker who negotiated the transition to open awareness when they could not do so (Glaser and Strauss (1965) and James (1986) report similar patterns). Both the Sister and the Nursing Officer reported that they saw this as an important part of their work.

Despite the difficulties of achieving open awareness all the qualified nurses indicated that they had developed strategies for 'telling' patients the truth about their terminality. Trainee nurses had also developed or anticipated strategies for coping with terminally ill patients although, as reported in other research, these were largely based on evasion. The following extract taken from the interview with the nurse with 20 years' nursing experience illustrates both categories well.

EW If the patient asks you outright if they're dying and you know then I think a student nurse or a pupil nurse might sort of hedge, 'Of course you're not going to. Ask the doctor'. But it depends, (. . .) Sister does allow us to use our own judgement, but just the same you've got to be very careful what you say.

DF Can you think of anyone you've actually told?

EW I've never actually said to someone, 'Yes, you are dying.'

DF But there are ways of saying, 'You're dying.'

EW I remember a lady saying, 'Well I'm not going to get better am I?' and then I said, 'Well no, I don't think so. But nobody knows for sure – if it's left to our care you will go home.'

DF So you always try to be positive?

EW Yes. You try to be positive as well because nobody can say, 'Yes you are going to die.' [She returns to this issue without prompting at the end of the interview.] I try not to lie or pretend to them. Try not to disguise. I try not to kid them along. I try not to say, 'Oh no, you're not going to die', try not to do that. That's wrong. They still need the same sort of – they still need nursing. It's just your approach to them. I think you should be as honest as you can. If you can't then I think you should get somebody else to talk to them who can be.

As these paired extracts show, important elements of the strategies developed were the need to be positive, and a stress on being honest with the dying patient.

EMOTIONAL INVOLVEMENT

One of the reasons suggested for preferring a closed awareness is that in such situations staff can maintain emotional distance from dying patients, although the evidence suggests that this doesn't work for nurses who have close contact with them (Gow 1982; Knight and Field 1981). Given the strong preference expressed by the nurses on Ward 6 for open awareness it is perhaps not surprising that nearly all of them (14) said that they were or had been emotionally involved with dying patients, often to the extent of crying and grieving at their deaths. All of the qualified staff and five of the trainees felt that such involvement was inevitable and unavoidable. For the qualified nurses such involvement was not seen as particularly problematic, and five felt that it was positively beneficial and rewarding for them. Trainees were not as positive, with four expressing problems arising from such involvement.

The following extracts illustrate the nurses' accounts of their emotional involvement with dying patients.

DF Is that a problem of getting involved too closely perhaps?

SD I don't think it's a problem, really. I feel that it's unavoidable. If you're keen on looking after people you'll be involved with them . . . If it's about their son or daughter or their home you can't switch off and say, 'I don't want to hear about that. I want to know where your pain is.' You *are* involved with them. You're their only contact . . . you're the only person they've got to talk to. They tell you everything. So, so you know them.

This student nurse had just given a very full account of her experience of nursing an 80-year-old terminally ill woman with whom she had become very emotionally involved. The woman had died two weeks prior to the interview and the student had shared the death with the woman's husband. Both of them had cried after the death.

> SH   Well, I shouldn't really have done that. I shouldn't have got involved so much probably, but it's hard to draw the line, particularly with someone like her. She was so kind to everybody. And I thought, 'Well, this isn't a very good example for the younger nurses, walking out crying with the husband', but I thought, 'Well obviously they know it's an upsetting thing even though they weren't involved.' And some of them said afterwards they were glad they weren't involved because it would have made them cry. But I wasn't the only one in tears so I didn't feel so bad. It wasn't as if it was just me who was involved with her.
>
> DF   Do you feel it is bad to cry when a patient's died?
>
> SH   Not really. Not if the relative's there and – he said to me then 'She wasn't just another lady was she?' 'No', I said, 'none of them are. Everybody's an individual here.'

In the next extract the nurse explicitly links the inevitability of becoming emotionally involved with patients to the use of the nursing process.

> DF   Do you ever find yourself getting involved emotionally with any of the dying patients?
>
> EY   Yes, I should think you get involved with all patients. I know when you start your nursing they say to you, 'Oh don't get involved with patients', but I think it's difficult to nurse someone if you're not really getting to know them. And when in fact we do the nursing

process here everything's a lot more personal. We're on first-name terms with a patient, so you do get to know them as people really, rather than just one who's stuck in that bed there.

Another indicator of the high level of emotional involvement which these nurses seemed to have with their dying patients was the contact which some of them maintained with the relatives of patients who had died and with long-term terminally ill patients who had been discharged. The most dramatic example of such behaviour was provided by the Sister. She told DF that she kept in contact with many relatives even though she didn't always want to do so.

> *CK* (. . .) Because often they are a terrific drain. And very often – you want to forget about work and it's forced upon you. I always have this terrible feeling that they expect so much of nurses, that you are representing every nurse. So to be unkind or to be curt, or not to have time would, well, have a devastating effect on them. They feel they could be next. And so you're obligated to give them every consideration, and yet I don't always want to (. . .) and I think that possibly the only common denominator with all these people is that they want to talk about their deceased. I have known them, probably in quite an intimate way. You can't nurse a dying patient without – well you *can*, but obviously it isn't desirable to keep them at a distance – and so you do get to know them very well. And this is what they're really after. They want to talk about the person, not the death (. . .) I can never bring myself to cut them off, and they may not be able to do this with anyone else.

Not all the nurses were asked about this type of behaviour as it was an unexpected topic which emerged from the interviews. Certainly the Sister was atypical in the extent and duration of her contacts, but four of the qualified staff and one student nurse reported acting in this manner (usually unprompted), although not necessarily over long periods of time. It seems that nursing a dying patient in an involved way meant that the nurse also became involved with the patient's relatives who often needed support after the patient had died.

A final indicator of the high level of involvement with dying patients can be seen in the 'adoption' of some long-stay dying patients into the 'ward family'. At the time of the research there was an elderly lady on the ward who had been 'adopted' in this way. She was, it seemed, the latest in a series of such patients to be treated by the staff 'as family'.

> RI (. . .) She (D) is like part of the family now, very much like C got to be in the end. (. . .) Sister's already started arrangements for – I know it might sound morbid – but she's told the administration we want a proper funeral, because D's got the money to pay for it and as many of us want to attend as possible.
>
> DF Is that unusual, do you think, for the ward to get that involved with a patient?
>
> RI Not if they're that long-term. We don't usually get patients *that* long-term. We had C because he was under 60 and couldn't go to geriatrics. There was no place for him. And we kept D because she was another one that was only expected to last a few weeks, and we all got to love her, and Sister K said it wasn't fair to send her to geriatrics where she wouldn't receive quite so much care. So – I don't think anyone can help getting involved though.

When D finally died the funeral was held as planned, complete with flowers, Sister K playing the organ, and with most of the nurses attending the service.

The involvement of nurses with their patients seems to account for another unexpected finding. Five of the qualified nurses and four of the trainee nurses seemed to be suggesting that there was no essential difference between nursing dying and other patients.

> RP Whether a patient's dying or not if they have an unpleasant smell about them they're harder to nurse.
>
> ER (. . .) People who are dying – we don't treat them any different, but I suppose (. . .) you get more satisfaction from sending some home well; we've healed them, better than sending someone home who is terminal, or

have somebody die in hospital. But you wouldn't notice any difference in our attitudes towards them.

One nurse even went so far as to say that she got pleasure from nursing dying patients.

> *DF* You said you got pleasure from nursing the dying patient.
>
> *EW* Well, well perhaps that's the wrong thing – *satisfaction*, I don't mean pleasure: satisfaction. You can *see* results from nursing a patient that's a long-term patient or dying. You can see what you're doing for them (. . .) You can make time to sit and talk with them. And obviously if they're dying the physical condition is going to deteriorate so you've got to be that bit careful keeping them clean and comfortable. Bathing and things like that. And to me that's nursing.

This was unexpected because the 'received wisdom' has been that far from being the same as nursing other patients, nursing those who are dying *is* seen to be more stressful and difficult by nurses. On probing it became clear that what the nurses were saying was that there was no real difference as far as their relationships with patients were concerned, although the practical nursing care of dying patients might be different, and in certain areas (e.g. diet) routines might be relaxed. While nursing dying people could arouse strong emotions and pose difficulties, it seems that it could also be satisfying for these nurses because it allowed them to implement fully their ideal of nursing care.

DEALING WITH RELATIVES

While the nurses, especially the qualified nurses, presented a generally positive picture of their dealings with the terminally ill, they reported much greater difficulty in their dealings with the relatives of the terminally ill. Seven of the nine trainees reported or expected difficulty in talking with relatives, with the two exceptions being the two student nurses who already possessed a qualification in psychiatric nursing. Four of the qualified staff reported such difficulties also. Basically the nurses' problems lay in knowing what to say to the relatives.

DF Anything you find particularly difficult? You said 'knowing what to say to him'.

SH That's right. You sort of say, 'Oh, I'm very sorry, she's died', but after that you can't just take them away for a cup of tea and say, 'Well, I'll leave you here for a minute.' You've got to be able to say something to relatives. You can't just walk out and say, 'Well, she's died. I'm sorry about it. Bye-bye.'

Two main areas of difficulty were reported: difficulty in 'breaking the news', and the failure of relatives to accept the news. Both qualified and trainee nurses reported difficulty in 'breaking the news', although unsurprisingly the latter seemed to have greater difficulty than qualified nurses, or were anticipating that they would find telling relatives about the patient's terminal prognosis difficult.

SD It's very difficult, I would imagine. If you've got a wife who comes in and you are the person that's got to say, 'Well, he's very poorly' and they say, 'Well, how poorly?' You can't say, 'He's going to die', but you've got to get through to them that they may not get any better; that they may not come out. You don't want to be brutal, but you don't want to give them false hopes.

Even when relatives had been told, they would not always accept that their relative was terminally ill. Such denial could, it was reported, create difficulties for the nurse in relating to the patient because in such a situation the nurse could not easily lead the patients to recognize or accept their impending death. More commonly nurses reported that while the patients would accept their condition their relatives would not do so. The following extract illustrates both of these aspects. It develops from the discussion of a patient with whom the nurse had become involved.

DF Is it upsetting to you because of what it means to *her*, or is it more than that do you think?

ER It's not really the patients, because they take it, they accept the fact. It's the relatives. They think, 'Why is it happening to my wife? Why this family? She's only 30. What about the baby? Whereas the lady in question, she accepted it very well. It's the relatives that I find difficult to cope with.

DF   Do you have a lot to do with relatives?

ER   Yes (. . .) If a patient of mine dies I see the relatives.
It's far easier to cope with a patient that's dying and
knows that they are dying. They've accepted the fact,
you've accepted the fact, and you feel quite happy
looking after them. It's the relatives that don't accept it
and are difficult. They do accept it eventually but it's
very difficult at the *time* for the patient's relatives to
think that actually 'He's gone.' I think that afterwards
they *do* think that he's better off, but at the time –
especially wives because I think they don't know what
to do, they've nobody to rely on any more – that's
difficult.

Central to both types of difficulty was that whereas the nurses
felt they could offer the dying patient something positive they often
felt that they could offer nothing to the relative. In particular there
was nothing they could do to comfort them. Further, when dealing
with the patient nurses were in control of the situation, whereas
this was not the case with relatives. There was no easy way the
nurse could avoid telling them the bad news, although with the
patient they could say very little. Such views were widely shared
and were expressed by both the least and most experienced nurses.

SA   Well, I think with that particular patient I could have
got away without saying much, but with the daughter I
had to say something to comfort her but I couldn't
find the right words.

CK   The difficulty with the patients is when they say, 'Am
I going to die?' It is always easy to say to a patient
'You have a malignant disease, but we have this treatment to offer you.' Or, if we have no treatment to
offer them, that they needn't worry because we are
going to look after them. We will make sure there is
no pain (. . .) And so I always have something to offer
the patient. You have *nothing* to offer the relatives.
You're going to tell them their nearest and dearest are
going to die. And then what do you have to offer
them? Because it is an inescapable fact. You can let
them talk, and you can answer their questions. You
can support them as you go along. But you can't take

away the inevitability of the fact that the patient is going to die.

The strategies developed by the nurses for coping with relatives depended largely on their confidence that they could cope with such situations and were thus found mainly among the qualified nurses. However, the trainees had, at least prospectively, similar potential strategies which they were waiting to try out. An important common aspect of these strategies was 'listening' to the relatives and allowing them (or nudging them) to raise the topic.

DF Do you find any difficulty talking to relatives of dying patients?

RL I did at the beginning but I feel a lot easier now.

DF What do you think has changed?

RL Probably because I've spoken to more of them. Sometimes I find it's just best not to talk, just to listen to what they have to say. Sometimes they just don't want to talk. They just want somebody to listen to them . . . I just tend to let them lead the way and just console them really.

THE ORGANIZATION OF WORK AND NURSING THE DYING

The ethos of nursing care for dying people which was found on Ward 6 can be encapsulated in the nurses' view that 'patients shouldn't be left to die alone'. What emerges very clearly from the nurses' accounts of their experiences of nursing dying patients and of their attitudes towards such work is a consistent set of predispositions to act in particular ways, namely: to become emotionally involved with the patients they are nursing (and their relatives), especially if they are long-term patients; to disclose rather than to withhold information about dying when this is sought by the patient; to be honest in their dealings with patients and relatives; to accept individual responsibility for patients while working as part of a team; to help and support each other. In short there was a predisposition to provide 'total nursing care' for the 'whole person'. Whether these attitudes were translated into action it is impossible to say in the absence of systematic

observation of their work, although from DF's adventitious observations there is reason to believe that they were.

General medical wards differ from other wards in a number of
ways with respect to patient flow and rhythms of work, and with
respect to the characteristics of their patients. They are generally
geared towards less intensive therapeutic intervention than acute
surgical wards or specialist care units; their patient turnover is on
average lower with a concomitant longer stay; and their patients
are older. Patients are typically mature adults rather than children
or teenagers. Further, deaths are usually predictable to nursing
staff and relatively infrequent when compared with some other
settings. Most patients recover or are discharged in an improved
condition. Thus, nurses may have more extended contact with
patients and so have a greater chance to get to know them, and
are dealing with deaths which are less problematic and less
frequent than those on the acute surgical ward studied in the same
hospital. Still, the contrast between the two could scarcely be
sharper. On the surgical ward the care of dying patients was left
to the untrained auxiliaries and first-year trainee nurses; on Ward
6 it was shared by all nursing staff. Whereas on the surgical ward
nurses caring for dying patients received little support from other
(more senior) nurses, on Ward 6 the nurses supported and helped
each other and the Sister was always available to 'step in' and help
any nurse who was experiencing problems. The pattern of interaction described by the nurses on Ward 6 is unusual, and requires
explanation.

One explanation seems to lie in the organization of work on the
ward. The system of patient allocation combined with the use of
the nursing process on Ward 6 meant that nurses could obtain the
satisfaction accruing from seeing the direct effects of their nursing
work, something which would be harder to do under the more
traditional system of fragmented task allocation. In addition to
such satisfaction one could speculate that feelings of autonomy and
self-esteem were also enhanced, and that the pattern of work
generated involvement with long-term patients, and reinforced
caring dispositions which might erode under systems where
fragmented nursing tasks order the organization of work (Charles-
Edwards 1983). With specific reference to the nursing of dying
patients, the combination of patient allocation with the nursing
process meant that the nurse would find it difficult to avoid the

patient because he or she was unambiguously the responsibility of an individual nurse, rather than the general responsibility of all nurses. Thus the commonly reported pattern of withdrawal from the dying patient could not easily occur in Ward 6. Further, such 'enforced' contacts with dying people could lead to familiarity with death and an appreciation of the rewards which can be derived from terminal nursing care, and thus might lead to a breaking down of nurses' fears of death and dying.

DF   Have you talked to patients who have known they were dying?

ER   Yes, they tend to accept. Far more than the relatives. You can talk to them, have a normal conversation with them without worrying (. . .) It's quite easy – well, not to start with, obviously – you've got to get used to it. The first time it's quite difficult. I was quite shocked the first time that they'd taken the thought of dying so well (. . .) 'Oh, I want to go out', he said, 'for a few weeks and sort out my house and sort out my will, and get everything sorted out so when it happens I know everything's OK.' Well, I was quite surprised because I don't really think about death – what'll *I* do when *I* die? (. . .) yet he was quite set: 'Let's get it down before it happens so everything is left all right.' He was great.

Another vital element was the support of nurses for each other, and especially the supportive role of the Sister. Communicating with patients who are dying and actually revealing to them that they are dying is harder to do than to talk about, and the Sister played an important role in supporting and teaching her staff here.

In the next two chapters we will look at nurses working in two very different settings: coronary care and community nursing, and see how their experiences and attitudes compare with those expressed by the nurses on Ward 6. In Chapter seven we will examine the relationship between such attitudes and experiences and the organization of nursing work in order to address further the question of which features facilitate or frustrate the implementation of the caring predispositions identified above.

Chapter Five

'Death is no failure':
nursing the terminally ill on
a coronary care unit

This chapter is based on interviews with seventeen of the eighteen nurses working on the coronary care unit of Midland General Hospital, together with observation on the unit. The main period of study lasted from late October to late December 1983, with the last visit to the unit occurring in early 1984. We begin by considering those aspects of the functioning of the unit which seem especially relevant for the concerns of this work. These aspects relate to the organization and experience of *nursing* work and do not cover other aspects.

THE UNIT

The coronary care unit (CCU) at Midland General was one of several units serving the city. It differed from most CCUs in two important ways. First, it had an 'open plan' design rather than the more common design where each patient is nursed in a separate room with no view of other patients. Second, it did not admit patients via an accident and emergency unit. Patients arrived either directly as a result of general practitioner referrals or through emergency ambulance admissions. That is, unlike most CCUs there was no 'filtering' or 'vetting' of patients in the hospital to establish their suitability for admission to coronary care prior to their admission to the unit. Over half the admissions to the unit proved either not to have heart disease or to have heart disease in association with another condition which made them inappropriate for treatment on the unit. The unit had eight beds, six of them on the open-plan main unit and two in rooms with large glass windows looking onto the main unit. These windows

63

could be screened off with venetian blinds. Long-stay and/or more seriously ill patients were more likely to be put into these rooms. Average bed occupancy during 1983 was 6.5 beds per day (81 per cent).

On coronary care, as with Ward 6, there was not a great deal of emphasis on 'getting through the work' (Clarke 1978). The pattern of work on the unit differed from that on the wards in many ways, the most important of which related to the type of nursing work, and the flow of patients through the unit. Nursing work was more technical and 'medically oriented' than on the wards, involving a great deal of expertise on the heart and its (mal)functioning, monitor patterns, and drug use. The role of the nurse was consequently 'extended' beyond the normal respon-sibilities found on the wards and nurses were legally covered to administer drugs and to initiate life-saving actions in the absence of a doctor. The work was also more intermittent than on a ward. Some of the differences are neatly encapsulated in the following comparison of CCU work with this nurse's previous experience on a geriatric ward.

> RJ The pace is different. On geriatrics you tend to be busy
> all the time but the work's different. You're doing a lot
> of basic things for people that can't do it themselves
> like washing them and bathing them and taking them to
> the toilet, and that keeps you going pretty much all the
> time. You've also got a lot of relatives to deal with and
> patients tend to stay longer than they do on coronary
> care. On coronary care the patients are mostly quite fit,
> apart from the fact that they've had a heart attack so
> really we just concentrate on one aspect of the heart
> attack, rather than any other problems, because usually
> patients that have got a lot of problems aren't admitted
> to coronary care. The work load is more medically
> oriented rather than more socially on the ward.
> (. . .)
> It's not sort of *ordered* or routine but things get done
> if they need to get done, but if it's not important they
> might get left. Whereas on another ward things might
> have to be done by dinner time, it doesn't really matter
> if it's not done. Things get done that need to be done.

All of the regular nursing staff were qualified, and trainee nurses were not usually attached to the unit. Apart from the senior Sister who only worked days, the staff rotated through the two day shifts and the night shift. Thus, unlike the other wards, there was no separation between 'day' and 'night' staff. 'Charge nurse' responsibility was shared by all nurses who had qualified for 'cover' regardless of whether they were staff or enrolled nurses. All nurses were treated as equal partners within the work team, and each took responsibility for their own patients under the system of patient allocation which operated on the unit. The extra responsibility of the work, the 'extended' role of the nurse, and the atmosphere of the unit were all cited by various nurses as attractive aspects of the work. Enrolled nurses in particular seemed to see the first two as important. The senior Sister summarized a number of these aspects during her account of the unit.

> *CV* As far as the SENs are concerned I think they get treated equally with the staff nurses, and probably more equally than anywhere else. We have this thing called 'cover' so that they are covered to be in charge . . . to be safe. Basically to give I.V. drugs without a doctor being there, to initiate treatment etc. – and if an SEN is on and they've been covered longer, then they're in charge. And there's no 'yes' or 'no' about it. So they're totally treated as an equal. A lot of them find that they need longer before they'll take their cover, because of the confidence thing – 'My God, can I really be in charge over staff nurses?' I think that's one of the main reasons why SENs stay longer, because they have far more responsibility here. They just get to do more. They get trusted more. And allowed to think.

A view confirmed by this enrolled nurse.

> *DF* What do you like about the unit?
>
> *ET* It's your responsibility as a person. You work your own routine out, whereas it's not set like a ward. You've got experience in the fact that that you're doing things that you wouldn't normally do on a ward, like taking blood, doing ECGs, which is very interesting

> . . . And no two patients are the same; even with the
> same heart attack no two patients will react the same.

The most obvious characteristic of patient flow through the unit was its great variability. There was apparently a seasonal variation to patient flow, with the greater volume of work during the winter months. However, there was also a large amount of variation from day to day, and hour to hour. Indeed the tempo of work could drastically change in minutes with the admission of new patients. DF witnessed days when only two beds were occupied during his stay and others when seven beds were filled at the start and end of his visit, but with three or four discharges and then new admissions during the day. This unpredictable pattern of patient flow clearly affected nursing work significantly. When the unit was 'empty' there was little to be done, and nurses could get bored. When it was full then they could be very busy, and have no time to take breaks. It was not merely the number of patients on the unit but also their condition which affected nursing work: very ill patients were much more work than those with a 'simple myocardial infarction'.

Patients admitted to coronary care were typically younger than those admitted to the medical ward, more likely to be male, and, as noted earlier, to be 'fitter'. Most patients stayed on the unit for 24 to 48 hours before being discharged to a ward prior to eventual discharge home. A few stayed longer, and it was this group of terminally ill patients which provides the main focus for this chapter. Few patients actually died on the unit (7.5 per cent of admissions in 1983), although some would die on the ward or at home after discharge from the CCU.

WORKING ON THE UNIT

All of the nurses had a very positive attitude towards working on the unit. Among the reasons given for this were their autonomy, the discretion they were allowed to exercise in the way they did their work, and the responsibility of such work; the appeal of demanding specialist 'medico-technological' work; and the relaxed atmosphere on the unit. In particular the good working relationships and informal atmosphere were universally agreed to be of central importance.

The 'sentimental order' of the unit (Glaser and Strauss 1965) was an important feature of its organization, and was something which nurses were both aware of and concerned to maintain. The main features identified by the nurses were their view of the unit as a team, good doctor–nurse relations, the responsibility given to nurses, and the good atmosphere on the unit. They seemed to make the effort to maintain a friendly, open, supportive, 'family' atmosphere which included *all* members of the unit, nurses, doctors, patients, cleaners, and ward clerks. A number of the nurses commented on the atmosphere of the unit, usually comparing it favourably with that found elsewhere.

DF   What do you particularly like about working on the unit?

RN   I like the more informal atmosphere that seems to exist. I don't know why that should be but specialized units, and certainly coronary care units, seem to have a more relaxed atmosphere than the traditional ward situation, both between staff, and between staff and patients. I think on this unit that's consciously created to some degree. I think we go out of our way to try and cultivate a sort of ambience because we realize that it must be a frightening experience for the people who come in here. Finding themselves in a place that looks like Apollo mission control, *knowing* that they wouldn't be there unless their lives were in danger. I think that the more you can take the stress out of that situation the better it is for them. You can keep the lines of communication open.

The maintenance of a relaxed and informal atmosphere and organization of work, where nurses were valued and treated as individuals capable of making decisions sometimes, it seems, clashed with sustaining a high level of professional care at all times. While the nurses were generally satisfied with their standards of nursing care, there were some reservations expressed by a few of them, who felt that at times standards suffered.

RQ   (. . .) we are a relaxed unit but in some cases I think we're too relaxed and little things like reminding them [patients] to take deep breaths and explaining why they

> shouldn't have their legs crossed in bed, and [RQ goes
> on to give further examples] . . .
>> The nursing staff should have a laugh and a giggle.
>> It's for our morale as well as the patients *but* there is a
>> point where you have to draw the line (. . .)

Within the general ambience of the unit there were changes of
mood relating to the pattern, intensity, and nature of the work.
Several nurses commented that the 'feel' of the unit depended in
part on the patients who were on the unit at any one time, both
in terms of their personalities and their disease conditions. On one
occasion the unit had filled up with elderly patients who were all
simple cases requiring little skilled attention. The nurses seemed to
be bored, complained about the 'geriatric cases', and were
generally rather 'flat' and lacking in their usual vitality. It was one
of those days when

> *ES* (. . .) nobody gets neglected as far as you don't get
> pressure sores or anything, but I do think care does go
> downhill sometimes. Especially if you're not busy. If
> you're busy everything gets done. But like today, it's
> all bitty and bobby really.
> *DF* Is that the problem, the discontinuity in the pattern of
> work?
> *ES* I think it is. But there's nothing you can do about it.
> But I think that must be it. I mean some days you
> can sit there and drink coffee till ten, then you can't
> be bothered to do anything.

By contrast to this situation, on the day following a successfully
treated cardiac arrest the atmosphere on the unit was noticeably
elevated, with nurses smiling and lively, and with a lot of banter
between them and the patients. A death, or the recognition that
a patient had entered the 'last days', could lead to nurses being
quieter and more introspective for a while.

The attention by unit staff to a wide definition of patient care
was emphasized by a number of the nurses.

> *CY* I think there's more emphasis paid on the patient here.
> If I go back to where I worked or if I go to visit other
> coronary care units the emphasis is basically on the
> equipment. The monitor pattern, the ECGs, their

enzymes, things like this. And although it would be untrue to say that the patient doesn't have a place it's not the main component. The doctor's diagnosis and everything is centred round the medical aspects, while here the doctors have now come round to a – not a holistic approach – but more psychological, sociological effects of the patient and his family.

An important 'structural facilitator' which worked to maintain the special ambience of the unit and which allowed this emphasis on the importance of personal patient care to be implemented was the high nurse-to-patient ratio of the unit. Typically the early shift had five nurses on duty and the late and night shifts had three nurses on duty to care for a maximum of eight patients. This high ratio allowed nurses to spend more time with each patient than would be possible in a ward situation, and so to involve the patient in the unit atmosphere. DF observed that many of the nurses as they arrived on duty would go and talk to patients, and would spend a great deal of time during a shift simply talking to patients. Patients leaving the unit were also seen to make a special point of saying goodbye and thank you to 'their' nurse.

A final aspect to be considered here is the relationship between the nurses and physicians on the unit. This partly depended on the low level of nursing turnover, especially as compared with the other city CCUs which were reported to have an average length of stay for nursing staff of six months. Before two new appointments brought the nursing staff up to full complement immediately prior to and during the study period, all of the unit's nurses had been working there for over 15 months. Medical staffing was inevitably characterized by a higher rate of change as junior doctors rotated every three to six months. This caused some minor problems for nurses. The two consultants in charge of the unit had both been connected with it since it opened, and had established good working relationships with the nursing staff. Not only were relationships good socially, but nursing staff were consulted about patient care and their opinions were considered seriously.

> *ED* Because we're such a specialized unit plus quite a few people have been here for quite a long time our views are respected and we are listened to. On night duty when you've got junior medical staff, the nurses really

have to inform the houseman, senior houseman what goes on, sometimes the registrars. And the nice thing again is there's a good rapport with the senior medical staff. (. . .) We have no problem phoning the senior registrar – and they prefer to be called at two, three, four, in the morning or whatever – to say, 'We don't think the patient is being cared for how you would like', and they'll have a word with the medical staff and sort out what's what or sometimes just say, 'Well, do what the nurses say' sort of thing.

The mutual respect, trust, and friendliness between doctors and nurses, and indeed all team members, were pivotal to the maintenance of the relaxed and friendly atmosphere so valued by nurses.

DEATH ON THE UNIT

Having sketched in the parameters within which nursing terminally ill people took place let us briefly consider some aspects of such nursing work on the coronary care unit. Table 5.1 provides a rough indication of the topics covered in the interviews. These are slightly different from Ward 6 in that those areas where a clear consensus was present, such as the effect of patient age or the likelihood of death upon nurses' attitudes, were not addressed in any detail. We shall consider the nurses' accounts under the broad headings of death on the unit; coping with death; communication with dying patients; emotional involvement; and dealing with relatives.

The first point to make about nursing terminally ill people on a coronary care unit is that death is infrequent. During 1983 there were 59 deaths on the unit and, as far as DF could discern, only four deaths occurred during the study period. A number of patients who are discharged from the CCU to a ward or directly home die subsequently, and even though some nurses scanned the obituary columns of the local newspaper and information would filter back to the unit from other sources, it was impossible for them to keep track of all their former patients and their outcomes. A second preliminary point is that on the CCU the differences between dying and other patients were reported to be much more

Table 5.1 CCU nurses' responses to various topics related to nursing dying patients

Aspects of dying	
Death often a release (8)	8
Short duration of dying easier to cope with (10)	3
No difference between dying and other patients (10)	3
Patients usually know they are dying (15)	15
Death is not a failure (12)	12*
Awareness preferences (13)	
Open preferred	8
Closed preferred	3
Emotional involvement	
Involved with dying patients (15)	12
Problems from involvement (15)	4
Involvement unavoidable (15)	6
Involvement rewarding (15)	5
Communication	
Openness and honesty important (18)	15
Communication with dying patients problematic (10)	2
Communication with relatives problematic (15)	15

n = 17

Table refers to qualified nurses only. No nurse referred to all topics. The number referring to each topic is indicated parenthetically ( ).

* Seven nurses directly expressed this view and a further five implied it in their statements.

evident than on Ward 6. Not only were deaths relatively infrequent, but the nature and duration of nursing care to be given to dying and other patients differed greatly from other settings.

> *RM* It's very, very different because a non-dying patient is only going to be here 48 hours, and if everything goes according to plan then perhaps will only have a bit of pain for the first few hours. And if you could measure input, that would be very negligible. They spend most of their time eating and sleeping. A dying patient is rarely transferred, a dying patient's going to be here longer than 48 hours. You get to know them a lot better.

While some nurses did say that 'they're all treated exactly the same until they die or go' (ET), or suggested that there were no essential differences between nursing the terminally ill and other

71

types of patient, CCU nurses were much more likely to stress the greater amount of nursing time and care involved in nursing dying patients, and psychological differences.

> *CG* There is a difference, but I think your *care* is the same. You give them the same support. But their outlook is obviously going to be a lot different. A person who is going to go home is going to need support for when he gets home (. . .) they're going to lead as near a normal life as we can get them to live. Whereas if a patient is dying, you've got to make sure they get the spiritual support that they need from whatever religion they are. They might want to talk to you or to somebody about who's going to look after the family or something. It's much less a physical thing, somebody who is dying. It's more an emotional, psychological thing.

Two patterns of death (or dying trajectories; Glaser and Strauss 1965) were characteristic on the unit: 'quick deaths' resulting from cardiac arrest (heart attack), and 'slow deaths' resulting from chronic heart failure. It is this latter category which provides the main focus of discussion in this chapter since it is this type of dying which requires nurses (and doctors) to make choices and decisions over a period of time. Table 5.2 depicts the relation between potential problems and these two types.

Potentially all patients are candidates for the first category, although this risk diminishes rapidly. CCUs were established precisely to prevent such deaths by speedy, high-level, techno-medical intervention. Thus in such situations the nurses' efforts were focused on preventing death through the application of their specialized training in a crisis situation. This could be very satisfying and rewarding, especially when they were successful, which was usually the case.

> *DF* Do you find it difficult being on a unit where you can expect death?
>
> *ET* No. I find it very exhilarating in fact. You're always on your toes that if anybody does arrest you've got a team. Really it's so exciting in an aspect that we've got to get there and get that person back. I mean nine out of ten we do get back. If they're here in time. If

Table 5.2 Nursing the terminally ill on CCU

Potential problem area	Heart attack	Heart failure
Disclosing prognosis	–	+
Communicating with patient	–	+
Communicating with other staff	–	+
Ceasing active treatment	–	+
Emotional involvement with patient	–	+
Impact on other patients	+	–
Disclosing patient's prognosis or death to relative	+	+ (–)

Key: + More likely to be problematic; – less likely to be problematic.

they die in the ambulance and it takes them ten minutes to get here we haven't got a chance, although we do still try.

Problems for the nurses associated with quick deaths from an arrest were concerned with knowing when to stop heroic treatment, deflation and disappointment at failure, and, especially, breaking the news to the relatives.

RJ That was really sudden. Cardiac arrest. One minute they were on and basically all right. The next minute they've arrested and everybody's jumping on them. It's a lot quicker, and you haven't got time to talk to the relatives or prepare the patient or anything really (. . .) It's just not dignified dying with a heart attack. OK, I know you've got to do everything. That's why they're on the unit. There's no point in having a coronary care unit if you didn't. It's messy. Drips and things. This chap had a drain into his heart that leaked and there was blood everywhere, and blood all over the nurses. I think the worst bit is the moment when they've been trying for about 20 minutes or so and the doctor says, 'OK, let's call it a day.' That sort of gets to me sometimes 'cos you try and try and all of a sudden you

73

just stop, and the doctors walk out and you're left with
this body, with all tubes and drains and things and the
bed that's all messed up.

Some nurses expressed the view that such quick 'anonymous'
deaths were unsettling because there was no involvement with or
knowledge of the patient, although for others coronary care was a
good working place precisely because they were unlikely to become
involved with the terminally ill.

The terminally ill patient dying from chronic heart failure posed
a different set of problems all relating to their longer stay on the
unit. Such patients could stay on the unit for up to two weeks
before they either died or, more likely, transferred elsewhere to
die. Because they were on the unit longer the nurses got to know
them better than other patients, and so might become involved
with them with all the costs and benefits this entailed. Their death
could therefore prove to be more disturbing than that of a patient
who died of a cardiac arrest on admission. However, deaths from
chronic heart failure seemed to present fewer difficulties for the
nurses in their contacts with relatives. The senior Sister summed
up the comparative situation as follows:

CV They both have their problems. A quick death is
     emotionally disturbing because, well it's sad. They're
     there and suddenly [snaps fingers] they're gone. It's as
     quick as that, in a matter of seconds. And a cardiac
     arrest procedure's pretty horrible even in a slick situa-
     tion like this . . . [with chronic heart failure] if the
     decision is that the patient's quality of life is going to
     be very bad, should we allow them to live? Then that
     is the decision. And then carrying out the decision.
     We're so used to acting. To actually sit there is – you
     find we all start twitching around doing anything in
     sight.

Deciding whether chronically ill patients had entered the
terminal phase and when to discontinue active treatment, were
problematic and required discussion with, and sometimes persua-
sion of, medical staff. While the decision to cease active treatment
legally rested with the medical staff the nursing staff contributed
towards the decision, and as one nurse put it such decisions were

74

'often prompted by the nursing staff' (CG). The involvement by nurses in this decision making rested on a number of factors: nurses spent more time on the unit than anyone except the senior house officer and had more contact with patients than medical staff; they were more experienced than junior medical staff; and they had developed good relations with the consultants, who respected their opinions. The nurses felt that the consultants generally shared their views about the treatment of terminally ill people.

ED   There's good rapport between the nursing and medical
     staff, and medical staff are thinking very much about
     the patient rather than just curing the disease.
     Sometimes it goes a little too far but with some patients
     it's hard not to; you've gone so far it's hard to stop
     really. Of course there are a few cases like that but
     most of the time if we feel that the patients are better
     off left we will do.

CR   The doctors are only here for six months and then they
     move on, whereas the consultants are stuck with us and
     likewise we with them, so you develop a fairly close
     relationship. So you really know when an individual
     doctor is perhaps getting a little bit out of their depth,
     and because we're specialists we do know and we should
     know a lot of what's happening (. . .) We don't have
     the final say. It's a medical decision ultimately, but we
     do have some influence on it.

The points at which chronic heart failure become diagnosed as terminal and when the decision to discontinue active restorative treatment were taken did not always coincide. The latter was the area where nurses reported that disagreements with medical staff, especially junior house staff, were most likely to occur, with nurses arguing for 'palliative care' at an earlier stage. Again the senior sister put the positions well.

DF   What about decisions in the life and death situation?
     Say, not continuing to actively treat. Do you participate
     in that sort of decision?

CV   Yes. I don't know how to put it really, junior doctors
     are inexperienced and a lot of them find it extremely
     hard to make that sort of decision in the situation

where you're resuscitating. They don't know when to
stop, and some of them are actually relieved when you
turn round and say, 'Hey folks, I think this is a "no
go" area' (. . .) But often it's a joint decision again
(. . .)

DF What about the 'cooler decision'? Someone who is in
chronic heart failure?

CV There we have the problem. Time after time I really
want to say, 'Now folks, you don't really think that
this is a patient that needs to be resuscitated. Have
you looked at the quality of life of this patient?' 'Yes,
but . . .' 'Yes, but what? There is no failure in death.'
And sometimes you tend to get a lot of those sort of
patients all at once where there's a 'Should we?
Shouldn't we?' and I think that nurses tend to – I
don't mean give up – but tend to look at things from
that point of view earlier than the medical staff. We
see the relatives much more. We see the distress that
they are having, and the patient. And it is an
extremely difficult problem with advances in medical
treatment and it is getting worse.

The rapport with and support from the consultants were important for the resolution of disagreement with junior doctors, since
the consultants were reported usually to support the nurses' view.
This was described by a number of nurses, all of whom were
careful to say that such disagreements were infrequent, and that
they could usually be handled tactfully by the nurse. They were
also most likely to occur during the early stages of a junior
doctor's period of attachment to the unit. In the worst eventuality
nurses reported that they could and did telephone the consultant
for support, if need be at his home.

Deciding to discontinue treatment was difficult to accept, even
when it was obviously the correct choice. While nurses were
generally negative about unduly continuing active treatment for
the terminally ill and, as DF observed, expressed satisfaction when
the decision to cease treatment was made, it seems that some were
still uncomfortable with such decisions.

EK I told you about that chap we got very upset about,
and argued about [with the doctor] until the nurses got

together and made a decision and went above the
doctor . . . I realized he had been such a previously fit
man that if we did *scrape* him through and get him
home, then what was he going to be like, and how
long was he going to last, and was it really fair? But
either way – if you say, 'Oh, let this one go' or 'We'll
go all out to save this one' – either way you're making
a decision. But is it really a decision? Is it *ever* your
decision?

One way in which nurses alleviated such anxieties in cases of
treatable arrythmia was to utilize a 'one shock' decision rule. That
is, such patients, when their heart stopped, would be given an
electric shock or short series of shocks to restart the heart, but such
attempts would not be persisted with. It must be emphasised that
this decision rested with the medical staff, although the nurses
could greatly influence this decision.

> *RF* (. . .) perhaps sometimes we'll say, 'Oh, we'll give
> them one shock.' Supposing they are in their seventies
> and their health isn't too good and obviously the
> natural process has to happen sometime. Then perhaps
> you think of a minimum of intervention. Give them a
> chance of coming round on one shock or something,
> and say, 'Well, this person has got to die sometime'
> (. . .) It's a funny decision to have to make, but you
> look at the quality (of life) and realize that, well,
> they've got to go sometime.

If such a patient died then staff could say that they had, after all,
done everything possible. However, if the patient did survive this
could also cause problems.

> *ES* Then you think that you're just keeping her alive for
> your sake when she's so miserable and unhappy. I
> think she'd be better off if they did let her die next
> time. But she always comes round. They say, 'Oh,
> perhaps just shock her once', so they do and she
> survives it. And you feel sorry for her in the end
> because all she talks about is dying. She just wants to
> die. And you feel guilty then that you're doing what
> she doesn't want.

COPING WITH DEATH

Since the purpose of the unit was to prevent death, the possibility of death was to some extent a pervasive and inescapable part of the nurses' work. This being so it might have been expected that when death did occur, or when someone was defined as being in the terminal stages of their illness, this would be regarded by staff as some sort of 'failure'. However, this did not appear to be the case. The infrequency and the nature of death were clearly key features in the nurses' view that death was not a failure as far as they were concerned. The nurses felt that patients died because, quite literally, there was physically nothing more that staff could do for them.

> RN We're dealing with people on a fairly narrow range of
> medical problems and usually we *know* whether we can
> do anything constructive in a situation or whether it's
> hopeless, and so we're not left with that guilt feeling
> that I experienced sometimes as a student of not know-
> ing whether there might have been anything more that
> I could have done, because usually here you say,
> 'Well, we did everything that could possibly have been
> done in the situation and there was nothing I could
> have done to avert what happened.' So that's just the
> way it is.

Nurses seemed to find a patient's death much easier to cope with than junior house staff, many of whom – or so it was reported – did see death as a personal failure on their part, and who would try to continue aggressive treatment long after it was warranted. This is not to say that nurses failed to be upset by a death, merely that they seemed to have developed ways of accept-ing it. The main techniques which they reported using were denial, and the rationalizations that there was 'nothing more that could be done' and that death was not only inevitable but also a 'release' for the patient, who would have had a very poor quality of life if he or she had survived.

> DF You said sometimes you get upset when a patient dies.
> How do you cope with that?
> CG Um . . . Just try to bring oneself round to the fact
> that there was nothing more that medicine could do for

him, and that there was nothing more nursing-wise
we could have done anyway. He was comfortable,
accepted that he was dying. He didn't die alone and
he didn't die afraid. And I just remind myself of the
good bits of it. And that he died with dignity. I
don't think you can die with dignity if you are
afraid.

Glaser and Strauss (1965) also report this use of 'nothing more to
do' reasoning.

Closely associated with the view that death was not a failure,
was the view (also expressed on Ward 6) that death was often a
'release' for patients.

> *EA* (. . .) although most of the times when you do lose
> them they are better off. You know, not in any
> physical pain, there's not somebody doing something to
> them all the time . . . when the patient dies you're to
> some degree a lot more relieved.

Not all deaths were viewed with detachment or equanimity, nor
were all deaths seen as a 'release'. There were clearly some
'failures' – some patients whom a nurse might have felt should not
have died – but these seemed to be few and far between.

> *RQ* Some patients come in absolutely clapped out and the
> best thing for them is to die peacefully, as peacefully as
> possible. There's just going to be no way out for them.
> You can see that. You can feel that. You don't need
> to know the blood pressure or anything like that, you
> just *know* it. Then there is the patient who you've got
> to know and you feel that he has got a fighting chance,
> no matter how slim those chances are, and those are
> the ones that you're fighting for. And you encourage
> the patient to fight as much as possible as well. And
> those [pause] – I've not lost many like that, but there
> have been the one or two.

As this extract shows, cases of 'failure' were closely linked to the
idea that nurses are fighting with the patient against the disease.
Not all nurses expressed such a view, but there clearly was some
tension between the feelings of fighting to 'save' patients and

accepting that in some cases death was an inevitable outcome about which nothing could be done.

From this discussion of death and dying on the CCU it can be seen that nursing dying patients on the unit was different in a number of ways from nursing dying patients on acute surgical or general medical wards. Death is generally expected and relatively short term, and CCU nurses generally felt that everything which could have been done to prevent the death had been done. In such circumstances death was seen as not only inevitable but sometimes as a release for the terminally ill person. CCU deaths were not only largely unavoidable, they were also to a large extent predictable both in the sense that anyone could die, and in the more precise sense that the nurses could often predict *when* a patient was likely to die. There were, as one nurse put it, 'not many surprises' (RN). Because death was so rarely a genuine surprise for the nurses this also made it relatively easy to cope with. There was also apparently a lot of 'mutual leaning' (CR) and support for each other from team members. Also, it seems that the emphasis on 'caring nursing' which was such an important component of the units' ethos served as a counterbalance to the medico-technical, interventionist aspect of coronary care nursing work, and made it easier to accept death for those for whom 'everything had been done'.

COMMUNICATION WITH DYING PATIENTS

Most CCU nurses preferred the 'open awareness' context, and said that they found it easier talking with terminally ill patients if they were aware that they were dying. However, as on Ward 6, there seemed to be some difficulty in achieving this. The practical issues of what should be said to the patient, and when, how and by whom, had to be resolved for each case. As it is difficult to discuss these problems abstractly, we will begin with an extensive account about one terminally ill patient who was on the unit at the time of the study.

George was readmitted to the unit three days after his discharge from CCU to a ward and stayed on the unit for seven days before being discharged home. He was then readmitted again shortly before the end of the study period and subsequently died. DF noticed that George seemed to occupy more nursing time than

most other patients, and his research diary contains several notes
of nurses spending long periods of time attending to his physical
requirements or simply talking to him. RM's account was verified
on a number of points by George himself when he talked with DF.

DF   'You have enough time for the patient.' In what sense
     do you mean that?

RM   Well, initially I think it needs a lot of, not so much
     time with the patient, but a lot of discussion about the
     patient away from them and just deciding about how
     you are going to go about it so each of you is doing
     the same thing. But you need a lot of time just to
     answer questions, to devote a few hours to be able to
     do that.

DF   Have you spent literally a few hours with a dying
     patient talking to them about it?

RM   Yes. In fact the chap I'm looking after at the moment.
     You wouldn't call him a dying patient in the fact that
     he's not going to die in a couple of days, but he's
     spent the past few days coming to terms with the fact
     that he's a chronic illness and he is going to die and
     it could be his last breath. I suppose that the day
     before yesterday most of the shift I spent with him
     (. . .) He's the classic cardiac cripple who goes slowly.
     He just doesn't have much of a heart left.
       It's easy with George at the moment because he
     knows he is going to die, and it's all out in the open.
     So you don't have to mince words, but you do a little
     bit because he's not really – well, I think it's a rare
     occasion if someone really comes to terms with their
     own death. You still have to be very careful, but if
     it's out in the open it's easy and you know you're not
     going to upset him. Whereas if you are looking after
     somebody who is fighting for his life it's difficult to
     find the right point to – you know, you never give
     up. Rarely do people give up here. Nobody will take
     the responsibility to say 'That's it', but you always
     hope for that one chance. By saying to the chap
     'That's it' you might just contribute to their death by
     giving up themselves.

DF Who told George?

RM CV. Sometimes you don't have any choice, you can't decide who is going to tell them. Suddenly the situation is there and it's no good looking for the nurse that's looking after them or knows them best . . . each situation is individual and different from the last one, and you just can't have a set protocol or something. I mean the only protocol can be that as far as possible you tell the truth and a lot of tact and thought and you can't really do any harm.

He was very depressed and actually said, 'This is it isn't it?', and it was pretty straightforward. She said, 'Well, I don't think you are going to leave here, do you?' In fact he is. His death isn't really very long away. But we have a bit of problem with him in that I feel he thinks that somehow he's cheated death, and he's beating it. But really all that's happened is he's changed his state of mind. He's higher than he was; he's just not depressed.

(. . .) I just gave him the practical duties of getting through the day, and said, 'That's what you're concerned with. No matter what, those things have to keep going.' And I suppose you can in a way forget about the future if you concern yourself with a shave, and see what's going to happen after.

DF The other thing you were saying, that everybody involved with the patient was involved in the decision. That means both nurses *and* physicians?

RM With the time to tell? And how much telling it wants and the rest of it? [Yes] Usually, yes. Well, the ideal situation is that everybody knows what's going on. It has to be because sometimes it's a very subtle build-up. You introduce more information slowly and if somebody comes in, and has only got to say a little thing wrong, it messes the whole thing up. So everybody has to know what's going on.

This account exemplifies a number of themes and issues reported by other nurses. Namely, the relative ease of interaction when the patient knew; honesty in communication with dying patients; that discussion and communication with other unit staff was essential; that there could be no fixed way to inform patients of their terminal prognosis; the extended period of time over which such disclosure could take place; that disclosure was not a 'once and for all' event; and the belief that in some cases disclosure could lead to patients 'giving up'. There was an impressive amount of consensus about what should be done, but some variety in the nurses' accounts of the mode, ease, and timing of disclosure.

The strongly held view that one should be honest with the dying patient about his or her condition was perhaps most forcefully expressed by a third-year student working on the unit, although other nurses were equally explicit.

DF Did you have much to do in your training with people talking to you about nursing dying patients?

SU Oh yes, you're taught a lot at school how to go about looking after those patients, how to answer the difficult questions patients ask like, 'Am I dying?'. That's very difficult for a nurse to tell them that they are.
Generally a lot of nurses avoid that question, and don't answer them.

DF Do you find that happens in here?

SU No. Absolutely not here. I've been told the patient must know and should be told *exactly* what was happening, as must the relatives.

There was also agreement that everybody on the team should be kept informed of the decision to tell the dying person of his or her prognosis, and that if doctors did *not* wish such information to be conveyed to the patient they had to tell – and convince – the nursing staff of this fact. Yet while there was a general consensus that honesty and openness with those who were dying was the policy which should be followed, there were a range of views about what one *actually* did. Indeed it was often difficult to elicit anything more than rather general descriptions.

EK (. . .) We sit and talk with them, and give them cups of tea, and make sure they understand that there's not a great deal of hope. That sort of thing.

EC You fear that some patients might ask you if they're

going to die but don't really want you to tell them.
They want you to reassure them that they're not.

DF So what do you do?

EC Just answer their question really as best you can
without being too blunt.

One reason for the difficulty in specifying what one did was because, unlike George, there often wasn't *a time* at which a patient was 'told'. Several nurses stressed that communicating a terminal prognosis to the patient was something which occurred over time and as part of the continuing interaction and communication between nurse(s) and patient.

RN That's difficult to say because actually telling somebody
that they've got a terminal prognosis – it never comes
out in that sort of way. For a start people usually have
a good idea already so it never presents itself in that
stark form. People usually make it quite clear to you
that they *know* already, and so you're merely confirm-
ing for them something that they've already sussed out.
Or they make it quite clear to you that they don't
want to talk about it *and* they won't let you (. . .) I'm
conversing with people all day and the interchange of
information is going on all the time. I'm never sitting
down and giving them stark facts.

Clearly the high nurse-to-patient ratio allowed time for such gradual disclosure of prognosis and more nurse–patient contact than on Ward 6 or in other busy hospital settings.

Another difficulty was that there could be genuine clinical uncertainty about prognosis (hence, perhaps, the concern about premature disclosure leading to patients giving up). However, most nurses seemed reluctant to communicate terminal prognosis unambiguously to patients unless they were asked directly. Only three nurses recalled such an occurrence. Nurses felt that the terminally ill usually knew that they were dying whether they were told or not, but that not all of them wanted this fact confirmed (cf. McIntosh 1977). Further, as we have already noted, several of them felt that in certain cases informing the patient of his or her terminality could lead to the patient 'giving up', and three nurses gave examples of such an occurrence.

The open plan of the unit, the fact that patients were generally awake and alert, and the ease with which sound carried from behind closed curtains, meant that it was virtually inevitable that other patients would realize that something was seriously wrong when there was a death on the unit. Thus another potential problem for the nurses was the impact of a death upon the other patients in the unit. This became particularly difficuly if there were a number of deaths during a short period of time, since in such a situation patients would become very anxious.

> *EC* It's very difficult, I think, then to cope with the patients who are on the unit and have seen it all because they probably think they are going to be next. They've seen two or three people in the next beds dying, and they think that everybody on the unit is going to die.

The ways of dealing with such disturbance and anxiety were basically to spend time talking with the patients, and to be honest with them about what had happened. Again, some nurses indicated that they would only reveal the death to other patients if directly asked about it, and some seemed more concerned with distracting the patients. The following nurse indicates some of these tactics.

> *RQ* As far as possible we try to keep someone who is jolly and bright and happy on the unit and try and keep patients' minds *off* what is going on, wherever it might be going on. That, I think, is extremely important. But there again, I think that it is also important to go around and discuss with the other patients what has happened and find out – get the 'vibes' if you like – what that patient feels. Patients normally talk when that situation arises. They talk a lot, and you find out more than you probably knew before. And if they don't talk, then they should be talked to. Because they *know*. But to be told they might see it in a different light.
>
> *DF* So you don't try and hide it from them?
>
> *RQ* I don't. No.

There emerges quite clearly from the nurses' accounts of their communication about death and dying with patients in the unit a

85

tension between being open and revealing and the tempering of such behaviour in a number of ways. As we have seen a number of caveats were expressed as to why such full and complete disclosure should be softened, modified, or delayed. This tension perhaps reflects the difference between the theory and the practice of nursing dying patients on the unit.

EMOTIONAL INVOLVEMENT

One of the reasons which some of the nurses gave for enjoying their work on the unit was that it allowed them greater involvement with patients than was possible in other settings. With the high nurse-to-patient ratio and the system of patient allocation, the time spent with patients (even over the 24- to 48-hour length of stay which was typical) was sufficient for these nurses to become more involved with their patients than on a ward.

> *DF* What do you enjoy about it [working on a specialized unit]?
>
> *CG* Involvement. You can get more involved when you have a higher staff/patient ratio as you get in specialized units, which you don't get on the general wards. You've got 30-odd people to look after, that's a lot to remember all the little bits about them, and bits about their family, and just to keep the conversation going. Whereas here it's quite easy really. You get patients you really know pretty much all there is to know – or what they want you to know, anyway.

The question of whether nurses became 'emotionally involved' with dying patients did not seem to affect other aspects of their work with the terminally ill in a consistent manner. Perhaps one reason for this was the relatively short duration of contact which CCU nurses had with dying people, for even those people dying from chronic heart failure were only on the unit for a matter of days or weeks as compared with weeks or months on Ward 6. Another reason seems to lie in the nature of such involvement, which in most cases seemed to be contained and restricted to the duration of nursing work with the patient – a characteristic which does not seem peculiar to coronary care as it was also evident on Ward 6. This is well stated by the following nurse reflecting on her experience on a geriatric ward prior to coming to the unit.

> *RJ* (. . .) because it's only short-term involvement. It's not
> like your mum or dad or somebody that you're going
> to remember the rest of your life. I mean I've probably
> got emotionally involved with patients that I couldn't
> tell you their names now. But while they were alive
> and I was looking after them I was emotionally
> involved with them. But now it doesn't bother me, it
> doesn't matter anymore to me that they've died. They
> were more important to me when they were alive,
> really.

There was a positive association between becoming emotionally
involved and a preference for the 'open awareness' context for
nursing patients who were dying, and between emotional involvement and gaining satisfaction or reward from such nursing work.
Open awareness and emotional involvement were seen as satisfying because these nurses believed that patients who were aware
that they were dying were likely to accept their deaths and die
with dignity.

> *RF* (. . .) some deaths are quite pleasant, really. You know
> people who accept that they're going to die and get
> themselves sorted out and are ready to go. It wasn't so
> bad (. . .) you do talk as you are nursing them because
> they can do less and less for themselves, so your basic
> nursing comes in, which is nice because that's what
> you're trained to do. The actual basic thing, looking
> after people.

This extract also shows the other main reward from nursing dying
patients: that it gave the nurses the chance to provide 'basic nursing care' which they saw as an important aspect of their role. In
CCUs the majority of nursing work is of a specialized and
technical nature. Dying patients provided an opportunity for
nurses to exercise other, more fundamental nursing skills.

DEALING WITH RELATIVES

Nurses on the unit reported that dealing with the relatives of dying
patients was difficult. This was a unanimous view, and most

nurses identified the task of telling the relatives of the patient's death or terminal prognosis as one of the hardest, if not *the* hardest, aspect of nursing the terminally ill. Dealing with the relatives was invariably seen as harder than nursing dying patients, as the following short extracts show.

DF   What do you find particularly hard about nursing dying patients?

EA   Well, it's not so much the dying patients, really. It's the relatives. Trying to cope with the relatives mainly.

CY   The worst thing is telling the patient. Well, even worse than that is telling relatives actually – it is a difficult, distressing thing.

RN   It's people's relatives that give me the hardest time emotionally. It's the most devastating blow that anybody can receive and you've got to inflict it on somebody.

Both types of death ('quick' and 'slow') posed difficulties for nurses in their dealings with patients. The problems they identified concerned breaking the news to relatives, acceptance by relatives, and comforting and supporting them. All of these were generally felt to be harder where patients had died suddenly from an infarction.

EP   I think it's harder on the relatives when it is a sudden death. A long-term thing (. . .) she can get used to the fact that he's going to die because he's likely to be hospitalized, and she can learn to live without him bit by bit and slowly but surely (. . .) it's easier for them to handle because they half know, they half expect the patient to die. Whereas with a sudden death it must come as much more of a blow to the relatives and therefore it's not as easy to tell them. It's easier to say to a person, 'I'm sorry but he has just died' and they'll probably say, 'Yes, I knew he was going to. We all expected it and he knew too', and therefore a lot of pressure is instantly relieved. It's all out in the open. Everybody knows. Whereas with a guy who has just died from fatal arrhythmia, to say to somebody, 'I'm sorry he just died' . . . [*trails off*].

There was some division of labour between doctors and nurses about telling relatives the bad news, for although this was formally the province of the doctors it was often agreed that because of their greater contact with them, the nurses were more appropriate persons to break the news of terminal prognosis or death to relatives of patients in chronic heart failure. Conversely, doctors were more likely to inform relatives when a patient died immediately after admission to the unit.

RQ If the patients come on like that then I tend to be more involved in the patient and I rarely come in contact with the relatives. You know, always seem to be in the ward rather than discussing with relatives. The doctors have more rapport with relatives then because they want to know what happened; what caused the admission; what precipitated it. And they are better people to have a talk with the relatives after.

DF Do you see more of the relatives in the long-term situation?

RQ Uh-huh [agrees]. You really build up a relationship with them (. . .) I think the doctors are involved but they're more the outsiders because they don't know the relatives on a personal basis that we can judge the relatives. Sometimes it is far better for us to tell the relatives about the patient dying than the doctors because the doctors can be too clinical, dramatic, about it. And sometimes they forget that the relative is as much an individual as the patient they've been fighting for.

This division of labour was by no means strictly adhered to. For example, nurses would often have to telephone relatives at home to inform them of the patient's arrest or sudden death – a task they found hard to do. While the rapidity and unexpectedness (for the relative) of death as a result of a heart attack made it difficult to 'break the news' to relatives, when patients were dying from chronic heart failure this task became *comparatively* easier to do. Whatever the situation, it seemed that dealing with the relatives of those who were dying was potentially fraught with emotion. Patients were either unaware of their impending death (heart attack) or likely to recognize and hopefully come to accept it (heart failure). However, (as on Ward 6) relatives were reported as much less likely to accept a terminal prognosis than were patients. As with the patients, the general policy in dealing with relatives was to be open and honest in communication with them so as to keep them informed and prepared for the worst.

ED   (. . .) we try to put our emphasis on the relatives. We always make sure that they know as much as the patients. It helps make them – patients and relatives – feel at ease, that they know what's happening and that the nurses aren't keeping anything from them. It all helps to promote this more relaxed atmosphere and promotes trust in the nurses.

DF   Do you ever withhold information?

ED   Not really, I don't think. Sometimes over the telephone it's a bit hard to explain things, so you probably wait until they come in. You might say, 'Well, he didn't have a fantastic night' and explain things a bit better when they come in. But if somebody's very seriously ill you certainly say, 'His condition's deteriorated quite rapidly' or whatever. You don't hold those sorts of things back.

The main difficulty for the nurses in their dealings with the relatives of terminally ill patients was that while the nurses could assure themselves that they had done something to relieve the patient's pain and suffering, and perhaps even help him or her to a peaceful death, with the relatives such rewards were largely absent, and at the end, there was little or nothing the nurse could offer.

CR   Usually you don't have to say anything, they can see it written on your face. And that's the harrowing bit, when people burst into tears [*inaudible*] and there's damn-all you can do except give them a little bit of comfort.

SUMMARY

Nursing the terminally ill on a coronary care unit initially appears to be stressful and difficult because such a unit has been established in order to prevent death. Thus, one might assume that any death could be viewed as a failure of the unit, and would therefore pose problems for the staff. On the unit studied this certainly was not the case. What problems there were in relation to nursing dying people related primarily to those patients suffering long-term chronic heart failure. These problems clustered around disclosure to, awareness of, and communication with dying patients and their relatives. In particular they seemed to focus around the dilemma of translating what one should do into what one actually did. Even the most experienced of the nursing staff expressed this dilemma. No matter how desirable it might be thought, leading someone to the awareness that they were dying posed its own problems of management, just as maintaining a context of closed awareness did for nurses on Ward 7.

Chapter Six

'I never interfere with what they want': nursing terminally ill people at home

In England and Wales in 1984, 26 per cent of all deaths occurred in the deceased's own home (Office of Population Censuses and Surveys 1986a). Most people who die at home will have been admitted to hospital at least once during the last year of their life. For example 74 per cent of those in the Bowling and Cartwright study spent some time in hospital during their last year of life. Despite this, and despite the fact that most deaths occur in hospital, a large amount of terminal care takes place in the patients' own home (Bowling and Cartwright 1982:20). Hinton (1984) suggests the following advantages of dying at home: home deaths are more natural and the home provides psychological comfort by virtue of its familiarity; the dying person may have more opportunity to influence their quality of life; and they may feel more wanted by their family. He also suggests that bereavement may be coped with better if the bereaved have cared for those dying at home. The main disadvantages to home deaths are inadequate facilities for the care of those who are dying; difficulty in controlling distressing symptoms; and a lack of support for the main caregivers. The care of the terminally ill in the community is therefore a topic of serious concern, and Wilkes' (1965) comment that 'the district nursing service is essential to these patients' remains as valid now as it was in 1965.

This chapter is based on interviews with fourteen nurses attending a course at a local school of nursing in order to obtain the Certificate in District Nursing. Eight were already working as community nurses prior to attending the course, six of them as night nurses. The remaining nurses had previously worked in hospital settings, with the exception of the family planning nurse.

The interview data are supplemented by information obtained from an open-ended questionnaire on 'Nursing the terminally ill at home' which was administered four months prior to the commencement of interviewing. Five of the nurses interviewed had not at that time had any such experience and so did not complete the questionnaire, although by the time of interview all had nursed at least two terminally ill patients in the home (in no case was there a contradiction between a nurse's interview and questionnaire response). Given the disparate and unrepresentative nature of the group great caution must be exercised in interpreting the picture of community nursing of terminally ill patients presented by these respondents. The main aim of the chapter is to illuminate the nursing of such patients in hospital by drawing out similarities and differences between the two settings.

DIFFERENCES BETWEEN HOSPITAL AND COMMUNITY NURSING

The main differences between community and hospital nursing relate to the nature of place and territoriality in the two settings; the central role of relatives in the home; the isolation of the community nurse from a group of colleagues; the nature of nursing work; and the relationships between nurses, doctors, and clients.

The most obvious and central difference is the setting within which nursing work takes place, since where interaction between health care workers and their clients takes place has implications for the nature and control of such encounters. The 'active practitioner–passive client' relationship identified by Szasz and Hollender (1956) is typical of encounters between nurses and patients and their relatives in hospital settings. It is much less likely to occur in the home, where the relationships between nurses and patients and their relatives are likely to be more equal. To use Szasz and Hollender's term, relationships are likely to be, or become, those of 'mutual cooperation' in the management of the patient's condition, especially between the nurse and the relative(s) s/he relies upon to maintain patient care programmes.

Quite clearly it is very different for nurses, patients, and their relatives to be nursed at home, with a different pattern of benefits, problems, and costs to be found in the home from those found in hospitals (Hinton 1979). In the clinical setting of the hospital patients are dependent on nursing staff for their everyday care as well as for their specialist nursing care. Both patients and relatives are part of a much larger group of patients and visitors with whom the nurses have to deal within the constraints of organizational routines and competing demands. In their own homes patients, and especially their relatives, have much greater control over their lives and are dealing with an individual nurse on a one-to-one basis and on familiar territory.

> *RW* [At home] they're much more in control of how they run their lives. You have to negotiate with them how they want to do it; in hospital it's the other way around. You could almost set down a procedure for it in hospital, whereas in the home you play it by ear.

It is unsurprising, then, that relatives were reported by the nurses to be more relaxed and assertive in their own homes than in hospital settings.

While in both settings the nurse's role is concerned with and constrained by the requirements of the patient and the instructions of the doctor, in the community nurses typically work on their own rather than as a member of a group of nurses working together. Community nurses are both more isolated from their fellow health professionals and have potentially more autonomy and control over their work than hospital nurses. One consequence of this is that it makes them more vulnerable and sensitive to the demands and wishes of their patients and relatives, some of which may run counter to their professional beliefs and preferred actions. As one nurse put it:

> *CL* We have a unique role because we're almost a member of the family (. . .) It's the uniform and the role that's got you into that so therefore one wouldn't want to abuse that. I'm aware that it's a special position.

The nurse's relationship to the supervising physicians, who are unlikely to see their patients on a daily basis, is also different partly because of their less frequent contact with each other. Nurses usually have more intimate and detailed knowledge of their patients and their relatives and their problems than the physician, although it is the latter who has the authority to control the use of analgesics and other drugs and to disclose or withhold a terminal prognosis. Nurses reported difficulties with GPs in both of these areas and indicated that they wished that they had a greater capacity for decision making about these matters.

> *CT* We're just told what to give and obviously we give that amount. If the doctor is understanding he will say, 'Use your own discretion', but obviously you can only go so far otherwise you're breaking the law. I think we ought to be able to make more decisions. We have our own patients and we know their needs.

When difficulties are encountered in relation to nursing the terminally ill person the community nurses interviewed could not, as was the case with those on Ward 6 or the CCU, rely on the help and support of a like-minded group of colleagues in the immediate work environment. While such support could be forthcoming when the nurses returned to their 'home base' at the health centre it was by no means guaranteed. Nurses indicated that they did not receive much support from the older and more experienced district nurses, who would not discuss the topic with them.

> *RS* Where I've been working at the moment I get quite a lot of support, but it just depends who is on duty. The younger nurses tend to be more aware of the problem whereas the older nurses tend to have the older ideas that you don't discuss it and that the patient or the family doesn't want to discuss it in any event, and isn't it the doctor's job anyway?

In any case, as one nurse remarked, discussing problems associated with the care of dying patients with one's colleagues during the short time that they were all together was more likely to depress everyone than anything else: 'By the time you've finished everyone goes out with a long face' (CQ).

Another difference relates to the type of patient being nursed in the community. These are typically elderly people with relatively stable long-term chronic conditions, although for community night nurses a substantial proportion of their case loads are terminally ill (two of these nurses reported that they had each nursed well over 300 terminally ill patients during their community nursing career). The community nurses interviewed perceived distinct differences between their nursing of the chronically ill (the bulk of their work) and of the terminally ill. While for the former their aims were directed towards rehabilitation and enhancing the quality of life, for the latter relief of pain and psychological support for the relatives were their central concerns.

The rhythm of nursing work in the community is very different from that found in hospitals, being ordered not only by the nature of nursing work but also by the need to travel from one home to the next. This could cause problems for the nursing of dying patients by imposing constraints on the time which nurses could spend with them and their relatives.

> CU I find it harder as a night nurse – we cover a very big
> area in Market Town, about a 15-mile radius of the
> town – so we're getting everybody's terminal patients
> on. Some nights you can have as many as five four- or
> six-hourly diomorphs or pepedins or whatever. Now I
> find that more difficult because you know you have to
> clock watch; that they're all due, say, between 10 and
> 12, and if you've got one in Hamlet and one in River-
> side [15 miles apart – D.F.] you haven't the time.

Some of Bowling and Cartwright's respondents reported that the nursing care their dying spouse received 'was inadequate because it was hurried or infrequent' (1982:35).

Community day nurses seemed to have more flexibility in organizing their work than community night staff, probably due to a greater number of 'routine' chronic cases and fewer terminally ill patients on their lists. The following nurse, who came to the course directly from a general medical ward, commented on this and went on to say:

> RH Nurses on the ward never had enough time. There
> were the ward routines to get through and other types
> of patients to consider, and if you were seen sitting on
> a bed, that was considered as you were skiving out of
> your duties (. . .) On the district you are the person
> who talks to the patient and they respect you talking to
> them almost as much as doing the general duties for

them. They know that they can ask you if they know that you've got the time to talk to them. Some are bothered in case you haven't got the time but they'll always just sit down and try first. You know, start bringing up some conversation and then it'll start to pour out, and they really like you to just sit down and just have a chat.

A final area of difference to comment upon is the way in which the nursing process was used and regarded by community nurses. On Ward 6 and the CCU nursing work was organized through the use of the nursing process, which was valued and generally thought to work. However, acceptance of the nursing process by community nurses was reported to be unenthusiastic, and there were perceived inadequacies in the use of this method of organizing nursing work in the community. The nurses interviewed felt that the nursing process was a superior way of organizing nursing work ('If it's used properly') because it was seen to provide a clear plan of action to be followed with regard to each problem – clinical, psychological, and social. However, there was general agreement among them that there was resistance to its use by some of the older district nurses, who perceived the introduction of the nursing process as a challenge to their professional competence. Further, the process was not used at all by night staff.

RV It's only we who are doing the course and our practical nurse teachers who are using the process properly and setting out our problems and our goals. The others are just writing it down. They don't understand the true use of it. They think that there's a lot of writing (. . .) some of them think it's a waste of time. I don't because I can see the plans working.

It was not merely resistance by conservative nurses to new methods and ideas which accounted for the failure to implement the nursing process. Lack of staff numbers made it difficult to maintain the record-keeping, and as the notes were left in the home where patients and relatives could read them nurses felt they had to be very careful in what they wrote. With particular reference to dying patients, it was reported that it could be hard to specify in writing what needed to be communicated to other community nurses. These points are illustrated by the following two extracts.

RV The nursing process is supposed to be used in the community [but] it's not being used, which leads to disorganization. You go into a house and nobody knows exactly what care to give and what's been given and who's giving it and who's directly responsible, whereas in the hospital situation you've got very clearly defined rules. You all know what everybody else is doing.

DF Do you think that if it was used the nursing process is a better method of nursing?

RV Yes, I do. Providing you've got the number of staff then it's a super way of doing it. But it falls down badly when there isn't the staff to implement it because then it becomes a problem to get all your paperwork done as well as look after the patients.

CU I do think it does help but I don't think you can write everything down, and certainly you couldn't write everything down in a house with a terminal patient. You couldn't write down, 'Well, I think that she needs us to do this because of this that and the other.' I think a lot of the things that they actually tell you are the kind of *unwritten* things, and if you try and write down unwritten things they don't read the same (. . .) you can't make sense of it the way you want it to read, and when it's such a delicate thing as terminal care what they've said to you is very difficult to write down so that somebody can.

The net product of these differences between community and hospital nursing seemed to be that the district nurse group experienced their work as more fragmented and isolated than the hospital nurses interviewed. Consistency of care provided in the community was seen by a number of them to be problematic, and their relationship with other district nurses and physicians varied much more widely than those of the hospital nurses. Their nursing work also appeared to be characterized, at least along some important dimensions, by higher levels of uncertainty.

NURSING PEOPLE DYING AT HOME

Having looked at the general differences between community and hospital nursing we shall now focus on nursing people dying at home. Table 6.1 presents the nurses' responses to various features of nursing the terminally ill, as reported in the interviews and questionnaires, and shows the similarities and differences between this group and the hospital nurses. They are similar to the other two groups studied in their view that younger dying patients present greater psychological difficulties for them than older dying patients; in their expressed preference for 'open awareness'; and in their propensity to become involved with dying patients and to receive satisfaction from nursing them. Like the hospital nurses they also believe that terminally ill people usually know that they are dying even if they have not been made directly aware of their prognosis. However, this opinion is coupled with a belief that it is not part of their role to inform dying patients of their terminal prognosis, a task which is seen as falling within the province of the physician. This group of nurses also differs from hospital nurses in

Table 6.1 Nurses' responses to selected aspects of nursing terminally ill people at home

Aspects of dying	
Young terminally ill harder (13)	10
No difference between dying and other patients (14)	3
Patients usually know they are dying (14)	12
Pain control a problem	11
Awareness preferences	
Open awareness preferred	10
No preference	3
Emotional involvement	
Involved with dying patients	10
Problems from involvement	5
Involvement rewarding	9
Communication	
Problematic with dying patients	5
Problematic with relatives (13)	4
Disclosure not part of role (13)	11
Support service for nurses needed	8
n = 14	

The number referring to each topic is indicated parenthetically ( ) where it is greater than those concurring with the statement.

their emphasis on the importance of pain control; their consensus that the terminally ill are different from other patients to nurse; and their greater ease in dealing with relatives.

Both experienced community nurses and those entering the course directly from hospital work were agreed on the differences between nursing terminally ill people at home and nursing them in hospital. We have already noted that they felt that they should not presume upon their special status as visitors to the home, and that they perceived and allowed greater control to relatives of the terminally ill than it was possible for the relatives to exert in the hospital. Nurses were, after all, dependent on the continued help and cooperation of the relatives in their nursing work. They were thus careful not to upset relatives or to go against their wishes about the care of the dying person.

> CE I don't think that nurses who look after the terminally ill at home have any priority or prerogative of care. I think that that should be the relative's decision and I never interfere with what they want. If I go to somebody who is dying who's unconscious, if the relatives don't want me to touch them I never do. For instance, they don't always want you to turn them over and I don't always turn them over (. . .)

Another commonly reported difference was that the relatives of the terminally ill were more comfortable and relaxed at home than at the hospital. This may explain the greater ease which the nurses reported about their dealings with the relatives (of the four nurses reporting that they found relatives hard to cope with, two were directly from hospital nursing). Caring for the dying person at home, it was felt, allowed relatives to concern themselves only with the impending death without any additional complicating factors.

> CO (. . .) because people haven't got two sorts of things to come to terms with. They've not got to come into the institution and be 'proper', and then cope with their relatives amongst a lot of others. Those things have gone. They do have to cope with the fact that someone is dying, but they can probably do it much easier in their own environment.

This does not mean that relatives and nurses had no problems.

100

For the nurse recurring problems were that many relatives would not accept the impending death or would not allow the dying person to be told that he or she was dying. In these situations especially psychological support and counselling were seen to be important aspects of the nurse's role. Indeed, apart from pain control, support of the relative was mentioned most frequently as an important part of their role in relation to nursing terminally ill patients.

DF What do you see as being the role of the District Nurse in the care of the dying?

CI Supportive role mainly. Ensuring that the patient is comfortable and has a dignified death at home. I think being there for patients to be able to talk to and relatives to talk to. To know there's someone professional coming in every day or every other day that they can unburden their minds to if they want.

Another difference which seems to relate to the differences between hospital and community practices was the great emphasis placed by the community nurse group on pain control. This aspect was mentioned relatively infrequently by the hospital nurses, and rarely as being problematic. On the ward and the CCU pain control was 'taken as read': it was something which occurred routinely, automatically, and without difficulty except in exceptional cases. For the community nurse, by contrast, pain control was often a central problem which they often had to argue about with the GP in that 'often analgesia is not well enough considered or prescribed at home' (RS). Other studies also report pain control as an area of deficit for those dying at home (Bowling and Cartwright 1982; Cartwright et al. 1973; Hinton 1963, 1979; Twycross 1978; Ward 1974a; Wilkes 1965, 1984).

A final area of difference which seems related to the differing contexts of home and hospital is the nurses' perceptions of patients who were dying. Whereas at least some of the hospital nurses, and particularly those on Ward 6, affirmed that there was no essential difference between nursing terminally ill and other types of patients, only three of this group of nurses said this. The reason for this may be that the contrast between the terminally ill patients and chronically ill patients with relatively stable conditions is much

greater than the contrast between dying and other patients on a
general medical ward, or even on a coronary care unit.

> *CO* The majority of your work apart from the dying is the
> chronic long-term disabled in which case it's really a
> matter of providing aids and/or nursing care. But
> they're very static and usually you can put a large
> input in, decrease it, and then sort of have a
> maintenance input which can be very minimal (. . .)
> with the dying person you start off with a reasonably
> high input and that input becomes greater as time goes
> on. That input also changes (. . .) with your chronic
> long term, or even your short ones, you're not looking
> at the psychological thing so much. You are looking
> more at physical adaptations for the home, say, or
> physical things which are easy to obtain and for which
> the majority of the resources are geared. You've got
> plenty of resources and help groups and equipment
> available, and you can have them on and off your
> books in a relatively short space of time. But with the
> dying patient very often you're not sure how long the
> terminal phase is going to last [. . . and] all that time
> it requires a much higher input and you've got to
> sustain that input at level throughout, which is much
> more difficult.

AWARENESS, COMMUNICATION, AND
THE NURSE'S ROLE

The community nurses interviewed presented a picture of interactional and communication patterns with the terminally ill in their
own homes which was quite different from that reported by the
hospital nurses interviewed by the author. In many ways these
patterns were similar to those found in hospitals by the studies
reviewed in Chapter three where doctors prevent nurses revealing
terminal prognosis. However, here it was the relatives of the
terminally ill (rather than the doctors) who were the most powerful
agents constraining the development of an open awareness context
with the dying patient. As with nurses elsewhere, the community
nurses interviewed preferred to nurse terminally ill patients who

knew that they were dying (the three nurses who expressed no 'awareness preference' also noted that it was usually easier to nurse a person who was aware that their condition was terminal). However, by contrast to the two groups of hospital nurses interviewed this preference was hedged with a greater number of provisos and qualifiers. The preferred situation is expressed by the following two experienced community nurses.

> CU It doesn't really make any difference to me. I think perhaps it [open awareness] is easier because you're there for a longer time they'll talk about things. And the things people have spoken about when you're there for four hours are obviously completely different to what they're going to talk about if you're in for just half an hour.

> DF Is it easier to nurse a patient who knows than one who doesn't?

> RW Much easier. Because you don't have to be so guarded in what you're saying all the time. You can make suggestions and talk about things with a purpose rather than hedge all the time because the relatives said they didn't want them to know – you're not exactly sure what they do know and what they don't in those circumstances. Whereas if they're aware they're dying you can find out exactly what they know.

> DF You said that the relative may not want the patient to know. Do you come across that very often?

> RW Initially yes, but as the stage progresses usually the patients become aware that they're not improving and that the condition is deteriorating, and then you usually say to the relatives, 'Look, they are aware of what's going on' and things usually come into the open at that stage. Not always right at the beginning.

More typical accounts of what usually occurred are the following statements, both from nurses who did not see it as part of their role to disclose a terminal prognosis to the dying person.

> CE Some are told too late. For instance this chap of 40 last year. He was dying for a long time but he went into hospital and they didn't tell him he was dying in

hospital. He wasn't getting any better and his GP told him, but too late (. . .) he died very angry. It was dreadful for him and for his family (. . .)

That's hard [if they suspect] because they ask questions in a certain way so that you don't give them a truthful answer. The would never say, 'Am I dying?'. They always say, 'I am going to get better, aren't I?'

DF What do you say?

CE I say, 'What has the doctor said?' often in that situation, but sometimes I say, 'Yes.' I mean people look at you so desperately. They so desperately want you to say yes, and they know that they're dying but they don't want you to tell them. And often relatives don't want you to tell *them* that their loved ones are dying. They know but they just don't want you to.

RS I've been dealing with one particular patient for quite a time now and it's really been a horrible situation because she knows full well what's wrong with her and doesn't want – does want – I don't know: for a long time she wouldn't discuss things at all (. . .) you couldn't ask if the lump in her breast hurt her because she'd just say, 'Don't talk about it. I know it's there. I don't want to discuss it.' So for a long time it was rather difficult discussing anything; all conversations seemed to be leading down the same road and they'd have to stop. I was rather anxious that I was going to go one step too far one day (. . .) This particular day she just said that she knew there was no future for her and she was finding it very difficult to cope with. She'd always been in control of her life and it was horrible not to be in control anymore. If there was something she could do she'd be happy to do it. And she said she was continually finding herself involved with happy-go-lucky conversations with people talking about things that didn't matter. She was embarrassed because she felt people must realize she wasn't really bothered. She had one thought going round in her mind and that was all she could think about and she

was obsessed with it. And yet she still didn't mention
that the thought was that she was dying.

The central element shaping the difficulties which the
community nurses had in attaining a situation of open awareness
with their dying patients was that they met the relatives of the
dying patient on a one-to-one basis as a visitor to their homes.
Several nurses reported that relatives generally did *not* wish the
terminally ill to know that they were dying – a situation similar
to that reported by the hospital nurses. Given the generally long
duration of such nursing contact and the necessity for the nurse to
have the active support of the main carer in the home it would be
difficult, and possibly inadvisable, to inform the dying person of
their prognosis when the relative did not wish them to know.

DF Did you find relatives were resistant to people getting
to know?

CL In my cases, yes. Two of them didn't want their wives
to know, I think mainly because they couldn't cope
with it. It was obvious that their relationship was such
that it would be a bit too hard for them.

DF What were your inclinations in those situations?

CL I would accept that. I don't think you should go in
and cause great catharsis everywhere (. . .)

DF So basically your attitude is that you will go with the
relatives' wishes?

CL Yes, I think so. If I'd known the family a long time
and I'd been going in for a long time and I suspected
– and the GP was aware – that maybe it would be
better to say yes then I would favour it [disclosure].

For the nurse who wished to lead a dying patient to awareness
of their condition there was often another important constraint. It
was often hard to call upon a doctor to provide high-status
'medical legitimation' for such action, particularly as many (but
by no means all) GPs were reported not to approve of telling dying
patients their prognosis. Whereas in the two hospital settings
reported in Chapters four and five the doctors allowed nurses to
exercise their judgement in disclosing to patients the terminal
nature of their condition or in leading them to awareness, in the
community many GPs not only did not allow this but actively

discouraged it. From the nurses' accounts it is evident that this
caused difficulty for them in their work with the terminally ill.
(For reports on the attitudes and problems of GPs with respect to
community care of the terminally ill see Bowling and Cartwright
1982; Rosser and Maguire 1982; Still and Todd 1984; Wilkes
1965).

It was not merely the attitudes of GPs but also those of the
older, more conservative district nurses which caused frustration
for the younger nurses in their practical placements.

> *RB*   I have mainly watched the District Sister I have been
> working with. However, my main problem is knowing
> just how much truth should be told. This has been
> influenced by my hospital experience, where the ward
> sister told most patients their prognosis. From what I
> have seen/heard on the district it seems that the truth
> is often avoided unless the patient has been told in
> hospital. [Questionnaire reply]

It seems, on the basis of this very restricted sample, and from
limited contact with district nurses in other contexts, that a large
proportion of practising community nurses do not see disclosure to
the dying patient of the terminal nature of their condition as part
of their job. This contrasts markedly with the situation found on
the CCU and Ward 6, where most qualified nurses, especially
those with greater experience, saw this as part of their work.
Thus, there was little peer support from their more experienced
colleagues for community nurses who wished to 'open up' the
awareness of dying patients.

The nurses' own perceptions of their role were important. While
the hospital nurses accepted that, even though they found such a
task difficult, disclosure of a terminal prognosis could be part of
their role, most community nurses clearly defined this task as
outside their area of responsibility. None of the six who had
previously worked in the community who reported on this matter
said that they would inform a dying patient about his or her
terminal prognosis, although one said that he might lead them to
an awareness of their dying. This attitude was also found among
the district nurses interviewed by Cartwright *et al.* (1973). By
contrast, only one of those nurses who had come to the course
directly from hospital work said that she would not disclose a

terminal prognosis to patients, the other five saying that they would either disclose prognosis or lead the dying person to awareness of it.

Although the reluctance of these community nurses to disclose a terminal prognosis to a patient is indisputable, it must be asked whether such reluctance was entirely a result of the structural constraints arising from the arrangements of their nursing work identified above. There may be an attitudinal component to this reluctance which is age related. Dividing the nurses into two age groups revealed that all of the nurses aged 29 or older (mean age, 34.25) said that telling dying people about their terminal prognosis was not their responsibility. Only one of these would do so 'if the time was right'. By contrast, only one nurse aged 28 or less (mean age, 24.8) said that she would neither disclose nor lead the dying patient to awareness of his or her terminal condition. While the older nurses did not see disclosure as part of their role some of them did express the view that they *would* like to be able to tell patients of their impending deaths if they thought it would be appropriate. The dilemma of this group is captured by the 25-year-old charge nurse who felt that because of his role he could not disclose a terminal prognosis to the dying patient, but wished that he was allowed to do so. He had been talking to the author about two of his patients who became suspicious because their overt conditions – fractured femur, arthritis of the spine – were not consistent with their increasing physical deterioration.

CO (. . .) So I'm constrained as to what I can talk to him in his medical condition. He knew he was incontinent because he couldn't control his bowels, and he knew he was getting a large pressure sore and he couldn't feel it. He was told it was arthritis and for a while he was happy to oblige with arthritis but as he deteriorated he couldn't see how arthritis could be the sole cause.

DF What did you do?

CO What I did in that situation was to get the wife told and support the wife. As concerns the patient himself you go through a chronic dialogue: 'This is a chronic long-term disease. It very often gets worse before it gets better. It's going to take months to get better if it does at all, but it's usually a gradual period of

107

degeneration.' So you're sort of spelling a gloomy picture for them without actually telling them the true diagnosis.

DF   Are you trying to lead that man to the realization that he's probably dying?

CO   Not purposely, but I think he knows.

DF   What would you *like* to do?

CO   I would like to tell the patient. I would like to have the authority to be able to say, 'Yes, you've got such and such, let's talk about it.' It's not always possible (. . .) I went to the GP and I went to the hospital and I went to the wife and the daughter and the son and I couldn't get one of them to tell him, and the GP just wouldn't talk.

DF   If you'd been in the position where legally you could have told him would you have done that?

CO   Yes.

DF   Even though all these other people didn't want you to?

CO   Yes. I was extremely tempted to anyway. Really, I suppose it came back down to when I was on my general training it was accepted that nurses did not, and it was only doctors that told patients. So in the end that was the one factor which overrode everything else. I'd very much have like to have done.

The net result of the features discussed in this section was that nurses most usually conceded to the pressures from relatives and GPs and attempted to maintain a situation of 'closed awareness', with all the problems which that entails.

CONCLUDING COMMENTS

This chapter has focused primarily upon the differences between nursing dying patients in their own homes and nursing them in a hospital setting. As individuals the main differences between the community nurses and the qualified hospital nurses interviewed for this study is that the former are more reluctant to communicate a terminal prognosis to patients. Although this may be partly a function of age-related attitudes (as a group they were older than the hospital nurses), it is suggested that other factors were more important. These factors are the relative isolation of the nurses from a group of peers who would support them in their work with dying patients; lack of support from GPs to disclose a terminal prognosis to the dying patient; and their dependence on relatives for the success of their work.

Before closing this chapter it should be noted that the discussion has been about the placing of emphases and not about absolute statements of factual differences in practice between community and hospital nurses. In their interviews the experienced community nurses would both emphatically deny that they would consider disclosing terminality unless it was cleared by the GP or a relative and also recount cases where they had led patients to awareness of their dying and/or acted as intermediaries between patients who knew they were dying and relatives who were unaware of this and who did not wish them to be told that they were. They also reported evasion of questions, and difficult situations stemming from their inability and unwillingness to disclose terminal prognosis. It is perhaps unsurprising that when this group of nurses were asked whether they saw any need for a 'support service' for nurses who nursed the terminally ill they replied more affirmatively than the nurses on the coronary care unit.

Part Three

DISCUSSION

For better or worse the human condition is a condition of imperfect communication, and we solve our problems in society as best we can through recalcitrant and mystifying symbols that cause the problems we must solve if we are to act together at all.

H.D. Duncan, Introduction to Burke, *Permanence and Change*

The organization of nursing work and nursing people who are dying

This chapter draws together the themes running through the preceding accounts and attempts to specify the nature, shape, and influence of 'structural features' of nursing work as they impinge upon nursing dying patients, and to attempt the specification of their main influence upon nurses' experiences and interpretations. The main features bearing on the nursing of those who are dying, at least as they have emerged from the present study, are shown in Figure 7.1. This chapter will discuss these elements with reference to nursing of those people dying in hospitals. Community nursing will be referred to in a less systematic manner, primarily by way of comparison and elucidation. The problem of what structural features of nursing work support and enhance or, alternatively, restrict and constrain openness in communication with dying patients will also be addressed. Before considering these questions it will be useful to summarize briefly the findings of the previous chapters.

In Chapter three the salient findings were that the hierarchical organization of nursing work in the acute surgical ward, coupled with the rapid turnover of nursing staff, meant that the care of dying patients fell largely to young, inexperienced, and untrained nursing staff. These nurses received little support from more senior staff in their care of patients who were dying, and were not allowed to disclose terminal prognosis to their patients even should they have wished to do so. To cope with the problems of nursing dying people these nurses used a variety of strategies to limit or avoid their contact with them, and were aided in such strategies by the system of task allocation which organized nursing work on the ward. Another consequence of task allocation was that the

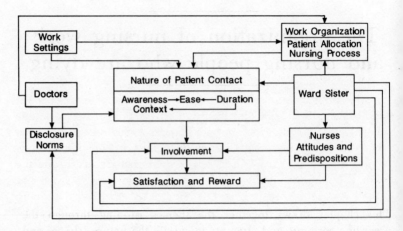

Figure 7.1 The organization of nursing work and nursing the dying

nurses were less likely to get to know patients well because of their limited contact with them, although this was less likely to apply to dying patients due to their longer stay on the ward. Nurses on Ward 7 felt that they should not become involved with dying patients, but were not always able to remain uninvolved. Despite the attempt by nursing and medical staff to maintain a situation of 'closed awareness' many dying patients discovered or suspected that they were dying as a result of the poor communication between staff which meant that they were receiving different messages about their condition from the staff caring for them.

In Chapter four a situation very different from the above was described. On Ward 6 care of dying patients, as with other nursing work, was shared by all nurses. The ward functioned with an overt philosophy of individualized patient care, work was organized by allocation of patients to individual nurses, and the 'nursing process' was accepted by the nurses as the basis for nursing work. Central to the ethos of the ward and to the care of dying people was the ward Sister's leadership. When nursing dying people, nurses reported that they preferred 'open awareness' with patients, but had difficulty in leading patients to such awareness. The ward Sister played an important role here in 'opening up' awareness. Nurses also reported that they became emotionally involved with their dying patients, that they regarded this as unavoidable, and that such involvement could be a positive feature for them in nursing those who were dying. This different approach to, and experience of, nursing dying patients seems to be directly connected to the differing organization of nursing work in this ward as compared with the situation described elsewhere.

The coronary care unit described in Chapter five presents yet another situation. The 'medico-technical' nature of its work, the short length of time which normal patients stayed on the unit, and the younger age of patients clearly distinguish it from Ward 6, yet it was similar to Ward 6 in its use of the nursing process, and the wide definition of nursing care. It differed from both Ward 6 and Ward 7 in its high nurse-to-patient ratio, the absence of training and unqualified nursing staff, the greatly extended role of the nursing staff, the absence of any separation between day and night staff, and its variable pattern of work. Death on the unit was infrequent, and dying patients were regarded as different from other patients in important ways. Possibly because of the clear-cut nature of what could be achieved to avoid death, and their feeling that everything which could be done to save life had been tried, CCU nurses did not regard death as a 'failure' on their part. They also seemed to become less involved with the terminally ill than nurses on Ward 6, and to view such involvement less positively. They did not, however, report the pattern of evasion and avoidance reported in the literature and found on Ward 7, but preferred openness and honesty in their communication with dying patients and their relatives. There was a tension between their expressed preference for openness and its implementation, with a marked reluctance on the part of some nurses to initiate or lead dying patients to a situation of open awareness.

In Chapter six the nursing care of people dying in the community was examined. The main difference between this setting and the hospital was, of course, that the dying were nursed in their own homes, and so the nurses were dependent upon relatives for help and cooperation in their nursing work. The bulk of this work was with chronically ill people from whom dying patients were seen to differ in the nature of the care they required. The nursing process was not in evidence as a tool for nursing care. Community nurses worked largely on their own, and with little support from others to lead people who were dying to an awareness of their fate. Although they might believe that an open awareness context was preferable for their work with dying patients they did not see the initiation of such awareness as part of their role. It seems that the autonomy of the community nurse was limited both by her reliance on relatives and by her difficulties with supervising GPs, both of whom usually favoured withholding the terminal prognosis from the dying patient. There was a difference between older nurses and those entering district nursing work: the former were more disposed towards disclosure of terminal prognosis and the use of the nursing process than the latter.

WORK SETTINGS

Some of the differences identified above can be attributed to differences in the settings within which nursing work took place. To specify precisely the grounds for such attribution can be, as the work of Strauss and his colleagues shows, very complex (Strauss *et al.* 1963, 1964, 1985). It is important to do so, however, for many of the difficulties which nurses experience in their nursing care of those who are dying relate to the structural conditions of their work (Benoliel 1983; Vachon 1987). It has already been noted that where dying takes place is an important variable. For example, in Chapter six it was noted that nurses' relationships with relatives of patients who were dying seemed to be influenced by whether the patient was nursed at home or in the hospital. One important variable between settings is the nature of 'normal' patients in each setting. On surgical wards and specialist units such as the CCU patients are likely to be young and acutely ill (sometimes chronically in the CCU), patient stay is short, 'recovery' and 'success' the norm, and turnover rapid. These characteristics suggest that little involvement would be likely to develop with patients, and that the focus of nursing work would be medico-technical rather than psycho-social. In these settings the dying patient is an anomaly – a possible 'failure' who stays longer than usual and challenges normal work routines and assumptions. In such contexts the dying patient could become problematic for nurses working with him or her. By contrast general medical wards are not geared towards intensive therapeutic intervention, and complete 'recovery' or 'cure' is less likely to be the goal of nursing work. Rather, the goals of alleviation of chronic disease

116

conditions and rehabilitation are likely to be more typical. Patients are older, and patient turnover is slower with concomitantly longer terms of stay. Contact with individual patients is thus more extended, and psycho-social aspects of care more evidently a component of normal nursing work. In such settings the long-term dying may be less of a problem for nurses and are less likely to be seen by them as differing sharply from other patients, as on Ward 6.

Individual and social characteristics of patients may influence nurses' role performance as many studies have shown. It has already been noted that nurses find nursing young dying patients more difficult to cope with emotionally than nursing elderly dying patients. Thus, the characteristics which are important to the care of dying people are not simply those related to a narrow definition of disease, but also relate to social and psychological aspects of patients as persons. For example, whether a patient is alert, confused, or comatose clearly affects the type of communication that the nurse can have with him or her. Kelly's review clearly demonstrates the importance of characteristics such as age, personality, and social background for the ways in which patients are treated by nurses (Kelly 1982). Dramatic examples of how social and personal characteristics of dying patients may affect the nursing care they receive are provided by Sudnow (1967) and by Strauss (1970).

Another relevant feature of work settings is the nature and level of staffing. The pace and intensity of work for nurses is not simply determined by patient characteristics, but is also greatly influenced by the number and training of nursing staff available to deliver such care. At its simplest this can be viewed in terms of the *time* which is available for nursing work. All of the settings studied seemed to be fairly well staffed, and so lack of labour was not a noticeable problem for them – a sharp contrast to the 'geriatric' setting upon which a number of interviewees had worked. However, the much higher nurse-to-patient ratio on the CCU meant that these nurses normally had more time to spend with patients, with the consequence that they could pay more attention to the psycho-social aspects of care, and did not feel swamped by more narrowly defined clinical tasks of physical care. On the CCU, then, staffing levels clearly enabled more time to be spent communicating with dying patients than in the other settings.

As has been noted in Chapter two a key element allowing hospices to deliver high quality care to people who are dying is their high staff-to-patient ratios. On general hospital wards around half of the nursing staff are untrained or training nurses whereas on specialist units and in the community they are virtually all qualified. On the wards there is inevitably a certain division of labour as a result of these differences in skill levels while in the latter settings all nurses are eligible to perform skilled work (although the division between 'first' and 'second' level nurses (United Kingdom Central Council 1986) can be crucial). Where there are training nurses some conflict between 'training' and 'service' requirements is likely, and as was seen this may be directly consequential in negative ways for the care of dying people.

The physical environment of the ward seems to be important also, for 'The design or shape of the physical environment in which patients receive nursing care appears to influence both the amount of time and the kind of contact between nurse and patient' (Walker 1982:408). Unfortunately the research methods used and, to a lesser extent, the study sites chosen in this work do not allow a direct assessment of this variable. Entry to hospital is a stressful event for patients, and the physical arrangement of wards and units may contribute to such stress (e.g. the comparison by a nurse of the CCU to 'Apollo control'). Unfamiliarity and stress may inhibit patients and relatives from seeking information or making demands on nursing staff, and this may become particularly problematic for the terminally ill if they are physically isolated in single rooms or side bays. In such cases their physical separation from the life of the ward or unit may become an important part of a process of 'social dying'.

It is argued below that regular contact with patients over a period of time leads to both greater ease in nurse–patient interaction with dying patients, better communications with them, and the greater likelihood of disclosure of terminality to them. The characteristics discussed above are important to our consideration of nursing care of people who are dying because of their influence upon the nature of patient contact which is found in different work settings. However, equally important is the way in which nursing work is organized within settings. Two apparently identical work sites may provide very different terminal care as a result of the different ways in which their nursing (and other) work is organized.

WORK ORGANIZATION

The organization of nursing work within each setting is another important influence on nurse–patient contact (Alexander 1984). The importance of work in this respect is well stated by James (1983:2):

> It is the 'work' of the unit which structures the ideals by which 'care' is practised. On the one hand 'work' consists partly of imposed events, tasks and routines which are to be accomplished, thereby fulfilling organizational needs, and on the other hand [it] is also subject to manipulation by the nurses. Since it is they who implement most of the 'work' – guided by ideals of 'care' – their interpretation of it and ways of carrying it out exercise a constant effect on ill-people through their relations with them.

Nursing work cannot be specified in all its details by others but involves a certain amount of individual decision making by nurses themselves about exactly how to perform their nursing tasks. The extent to which this is allowed, encouraged, or constrained by the nature of nursing work and its organization will vary from task to task and from setting to setting. In any setting there will be a number of work tasks which must be performed, such as giving injections and administering drugs, but the manner in which such tasks are performed may nevertheless vary quite markedly.

Nursing work can be construed as doing things *to* patients, or as working *with* patients. Most nursing work in most settings involves at least the potential for contact with patients on an interpersonal basis rather than simply relating to them as physical objects, hence it seems appropriate to define nursing work primarily in interpersonal terms, as in current definitions of good nursing practice in terms of individualized patient care (United Kingdom Central Council 1986). It is true that some tasks, such as those involved in dealing with a heart attack, will be so demanding that there is little room for individualized task performance, and everything stops until they are completed. At a less intense level the monitoring of machines may impose similar constraints. However, other tasks may be so routine that they can fit into ongoing nursing work quite easily, and these tasks will make up the bulk of nursing work in many settings. These are largely the invisible elements of nurses' caring work referred to in Chapter two. Such work as talking with dying and ill patients in the course of physical care may be both demanding and stressful *and* unrewarded and unnoticed by others. Further, because it is thought to be part of the 'natural' caring skills of females neither nurses nor others may pay much attention to care work as requiring skills which need to be learnt, developed, and supported (James 1986). It is perhaps instructive to compare the apparent neglect of 'emotion work' in nurse training with the training of airline attendants, where great emphasis is placed upon learning how to demonstrate care and concern to travellers (Hochschild 1983).

The method whereby nursing work is organized is possibly the most important factor influencing the ways in which nurses perform their roles. According to Pembrey, 'There is evidence that appropriate nursing . . . is related to individualised rather than non-individualised nursing. A number of studies describe non-individualised nursing linked to the failure to meet patients' needs' (1980:9). The nursing methods used on Ward 6 and the CCU seemed to contribute significantly to the nursing care of dying patients which was reported there. In both places teamwork and support were emphasized even through nurses were individually responsible for patients. Both Ward 6 and CCU were 'egalitarian', with the care of dying patients shared by all nursing staff, nurses supporting and helping each other, and with the Sister or Senior Sister always available to step in to help any nurse who was experiencing problems. As was suggested in Chapter four, the individualized system of patient allocation combined with the use of the nursing process on Ward 6 and the CCU meant that nurses could directly see the effect of their nursing work and so derive satisfaction from it. Where nursing work is organized along the more traditional method (allocating tasks to nurses on the basis of their status and/or experience) involvement and satisfaction deriving from the progress of patients seem less likely to develop to such an extent. Feelings of autonomy and self-esteem may also be enhanced for nurses who take direct responsibility for the total nursing care of their patients. On Ward 6 at least it seems that the pattern of work inescapably generated involvement with long-term patients, and it was suggested that it also reinforced caring dispositions which might otherwise erode under systems where fragmented nursing tasks structure work organization. With specific reference to the nursing of dying patients individualized methods of organizing nursing care will mean that nurses would find it difficult to avoid regular contact with the dying patient because they would be unambiguously responsible for that patient. Thus the commonly reported pattern of withdrawal from dying patients could not easily occur in Ward 6 or the CCU. The nurses' accounts from Ward 6 further suggest that such 'enforced' contacts with dying people can break down nurses' fear of death and dying by increasing their familiarity with death and so lead to greater ease in their interactions with dying people. It can also lead to an appreciation of the rewards which can be derived from terminal care nursing.

James (1983, 1986), in her study of nursing work in a hospice makes the useful analytic distinction between 'work' and 'care'. She notes the tensions created between the demands of work – defined in terms of finite and achievable nursing tasks – and the emphasis on patient-centred care, which was infinitely demanding and with no clear boundaries. The demands on the nurses stemming from their interpersonal care of dying people can be both stressful and demanding and therefore the fixed routines of doing physical nursing tasks, and especially comfort work, can be reassuring for nurses because they provide an important sense of visible achievement (Glaser and Strauss 1965; James 1986). This is so even in situations which emphasize psycho-social care as important, and so it must not be assumed that the routinization of nursing work is necessarily and inevitably undesirable. Physical work routines can be *both* restrictive *and* reassuring for nurses – and for patients – by providing them with structure and certainty. However, they may also provide a convenient escape for nurses from the demands of psycho-social care, particularly if they are nursing dying patients with little direction or support from other staff. The importance for the nursing care of dying patients of a system of work organization which provides help and support for the nurse in such work cannot be underestimated. For example in Chapter six community nurses were seen to have little support from colleagues and to report that they felt the need for such support. Vachon (1987) reports that team communication problems were the most frequently reported source of stress by her respondents, and that team support was the most frequently reported coping mechanism for dealing with stress.

Apart from the nature of the specific nursing tasks and the methods whereby work is organized, other constraints may be placed upon the nurse in her individual role performance. The skill level of the nurse has already been mentioned as another constraint upon her action. This refers not only to the formal level of nursing skills (SEN, SRN, and so on), but also to the nurse's confidence in her ability to perform specific tasks. For example in previous chapters it has been seen that nurses are not always confident of their general communication skills or their ability to 'lead' dying patients to an awareness of their impending death. This will be reviewed below, as will the attitudes and instructions of doctors, and the ways in which ward Sisters perform their roles.

DOCTOR–NURSE RELATIONSHIPS

Doctors have not figured as central characters in this discussion, although it is quite evident that they are major actors in the dramas and routines which work with dying people entails. The central feature of relationships between doctors and nurses is that doctors control large areas of nursing work. They do this both directly through doctors' orders specifying clinically relevant nursing tasks associated with therapeutic intervention into and management of disease processes, and indirectly through their general instructions about nursing work. Restrictions on the nature of nurses' communication with dying patients are most likely to stem from the latter rather than the former type of control. Even where nurses exercise autonomy and responsibility for patient care it is likely to be of a limited nature, and within an ambit of activity embedded within and hedged by clinical control (Moloney 1986). Despite their numerically small numbers, senior hospital doctors exercise a great deal of control over nursing work, and nurses must negotiate the 'space' they require for the implementation of their work in the manner in which they wish to do it. Where they have a clearly defined and well-established expertise, as in specialist units, they are more likely to be able to shape their work to their own requirements than where their expertise is lower, as on general medical or surgical wards. Continuity of doctor–nurse relationships over time is also likely to lead to the development of greater autonomy for nurses, as can be seen from the accounts of the CCU and Ward 6, where nursing turnover was low. With respect to nursing dying patients doctors can figure either as inhibitors of the development of open awareness contexts in their nursing care, as on Ward 7 and for the community nurses, or they can allow nurses great autonomy and openness of communication in their care of dying people, as on Ward 6 and the CCU.

The division of labour between doctors and nurses is clearly crucial to the relationship between them. As has already been indicated in Chapter two this in important ways reflects and is reinforced by the general character of gender roles and relationships in our society. Nursing work is largely defined in terms of personal care of patients – working with people – whereas doctor work is largely defined in terms of clinical treatment and management – working on or in people. Nurses' work is, at least in principle, more all-encompassing than doctors' work. The terminology of Strauss *et al.* (1985) is useful to describe briefly the differing elements of nursing work. While nurses will perform discrete tasks associated with 'machine work' or 'safety work' assigned to them by doctors, these tasks are often embedded within ongoing 'comfort work' and 'sentimental work'. In particular, nurses are more likely to do the important 'articulation work' which relates the different areas of patient-centred activity. An example of such work is the pattern found on both Ward 6 and the CCU of a nurse 'dropping out' of the continuing ward round in order to explain to her patients what the doctors had said about them. Nurses are at the hub of patient-centred hospital work, but they often work without direct instructions or written orders from doctors. For example, Vachon (1987) reports the stress created by doctors for nurses working in intensive care units when the decision to cease active life support has been made but not put into written orders by doctors. She also reports that nurses had more stress problems than other health workers as a result of their perceived lack of control and authority at work. The extent to which nurses are constrained in their work performance by doctors is important for their terminal care work with dying people, and will contribute to the sense of satisfaction, worth, and identity which nurses develop and the quality of their care.

The attitudes of doctors and nurses to their work and about their respective roles are also important. We have already seen that an important element influencing the community nurses' care

123

of dying patients was their belief that disclosure of a terminal diagnosis to their dying patients was not part of their role. Most doctors and nurses accept and believe that doctors should give orders to nurses and control their nursing activity in general. Most nurses are, it seems, still 'traditionalizers' who are willing to accept a passive role in patient care. The 'professionalizers' in nursing schools and the Royal College of Nurses must first convince practising nurses of their need to exercise greater autonomy and decision making before they can persuade doctors to concede this to them. The high levels of nursing autonomy found on Ward 6 and the CCU seem at least in part to be related to the very aggressive style of the Nursing Officer running the unit and the firm belief of the Ward Sister on Ward 6 and of senior nursing staff on the CCU that there was a legitimate and indisputable basis for them to control their nursing work in the way which they as nurses thought best.

THE ROLE OF THE WARD SISTER

Given the initial focus of interest of the research reported in this book the role of the ward Sister (or senior Sister on CCU) was not targeted directly for investigation, although it became quite apparent that they were central to the nursing care which dying patients received on both Ward 6 and the CCU. The nurse performs a key coordinating function in hospitals by virtue of her position at the intersection of so many hospital activities and groups of other workers, and by her continuing contact with patients. The 'coordinator of coordinators' is unarguably the ward Sister. It is the ward Sister or charge nurse who has greatest contact with doctors in negotiating nursing work in relation to doctors' orders and who organizes and allocates work to nurses. S/he plays a key position in establishing and maintaining the 'sentimental order' or 'ward climate', as can be seen from the accounts of Ward 6 and the CCU.

One important role of the ward Sister or charge nurse is the training of future nurses. As indicated in Chapter two studies have found a discrepancy between what trainees are taught in the nursing schools and their experiences on the wards where they are frequently treated primarily as 'hands' to work with rather than as learners to be trained and educated. The importance of the ward

Sister as a role model and source of training cannot be over-stressed, yet few of them have had any special training in teaching students. Recent research into the role of the ward Sister has mainly focused upon ward learning climates, but there is agreement that 'good' learning climates are equally beneficial to patient care, and that the ward Sister is 'the person, above all, responsible for the climate of the ward' (Orton 1981:62). Orton sums up such a climate as 'a happy purposeful environment guided and regulated by a confident, considerate ward sister who led her staff and student within a team' (1981:45). Fretwell (1980) also emphasizes the key role of the Sister in providing good communication and information, negotiation, and teamwork. From the literature it seems that such ideal Sisters or charge nurses and good ward climates are rare. Both Ward 6 and the CCU approximate these rare situations, and therefore it must be emphasized that the findings reported in this work are from unrepresentative settings. The situations found by Bond (1983) and on Ward 7 appear to provide a better approximation of normal practice.

What are the key components of ward climate which the Sister or charge nurse so greatly determines? Orton (1981) identifies individual autonomy, the degree of structure imposed, rewards, and consideration, warmth and support as the key variables and links these to leadership style. On Ward 6 an 'employee-oriented' style enhanced the individual autonomy of nurses within a well-focused and supportive structure. This allowed nurses to gain satisfaction and reward from their nursing work with patients, and to be confident that when they experienced problems, as in nursing a dying patient, more senior staff would be on hand to help them. The Sister's strong belief in the use of the nursing process was another important element in the ethos of nursing care found on the ward. A similar situation was found on the CCU, where the structuring of work was to a much larger extent shaped by the medico-technical tasks of patient care. The apparently very high level of nurse morale and satisfaction in these settings seemed to be directly related to these factors. By contrast, morale – at least among junior nurses – was poor on Ward 7, and this was directly linked to the climate of the ward. Work here was fragmented, nurses were not supported by seniors, and satisfaction and reward seemed scarce.

The nursing care of dying people can be improved by general improvements in nursing standards which seem to be connected to the ways in which ward Sisters and charge nurses perform their coordinative role. The important principles of recognition of the patients as an individual and good communication are often more honoured in principle than in practice. The ward Sister plays a key role in the implementation of these principles by her control over information and work organization. For example, Melia (1982, 1987) identifies lack of information from senior nurses and the organization of nursing on the wards as the main source of difficulty experienced by student nurses in communicating with patients.

The autonomy of nurses from the doctor is another aspect which is greatly influenced by the ward Sister, for if they are deferential and meekly accepting of a medical definition of nursing work then other nurses can hardly act otherwise. Runciman found that the 'inability to challenge medically sanctioned routine and policy, and the perception of doctors as more powerful than nurses' was one of the problems which ward Sisters reported (1983:34). In her interview study, 'disagreeing with doctors' instructions' emerged as a problem for Sisters, and 'the main areas of conflict concerned the care of the terminally ill . . . and the care and [unnecessary] resuscitation of elderly patients' (1983:95). She also found that the Sisters had difficulty in speaking out and expressing doubt to medical colleagues. It is significant that on Ward 6 and the CCU such reluctance to challenge and negotiate the proposed care of dying patients was not evident, and that the nurses had a good deal of autonomy in their work.

DISCLOSURE NORMS

Disclosure norms, that is the conventions which exist in a work setting about the nature and type of information which is usually given to a patient, establish predispositions towards action, and may also impose direct constraints upon nurses' behaviour, as we have seen. They are central to the differences between settings which are reported in this work. On Ward 6 and the CCU disclosure and open awareness contexts were encouraged, and nurses did not *have* to consult the medical staff before they could tell patients they were dying. It would be very unlikely, however, that the general situation had *not* been discussed by nurses and doctors, and a joint decision reached. By contrast, on Ward 7 nurses were *forbidden* to disclose a terminal prognosis to a patient, even where they felt that this was desirable or necessary. In the community there were also very strong norms of non-disclosure. The greater ease of interaction with dying patients on Ward 6 and the CCU seems to flow directly from the disclosure norms in operation in these two settings. These disclosure rules themselves were firmly embedded in the method and organization of nursing work.

It could be argued that disclosure norms are the most important factors influencing how dying patients come to learn about their impending death. Such a view, however, must not obscure our appreciation of the complex interaction between the various elements in the organization of nursing work which affect the care of dying people. The attitudes and practices of staff are clearly intermeshed with such factors as work loads and work organization, as this chapter has attempted to show. Where disclosure norms are unclear and not shared by all staff members, ambiguity and uncertainty will pervade relationships with dying people. It is essential that all staff members in contact with the dying patient have the same information about what has been said to the person, when it was said, and, as far as possible, how it was said. This is vital in situations were openness is the preferred strategy for relating to dying patients. Even where the norm is to disclose information and there is good communication among staff it may be difficult for some nurses actually to do so. The advantages and disadvantages of disclosure have been reviewed in the introduction. A more extensive discussion can be found in Glaser and Strauss (1965, 1968).

NURSES' ATTITUDES AND PREDISPOSITIONS

Disclosure norms cannot be divorced from the more general attitudes and predispositions of nurses. How nurses view their work in general, and their nursing work with dying people in particular, interacts very powerfully with the structural factors which have been discussed above to shape their nursing care of those who are dying and what they are likely to say to such patients about their terminal condition. These personal attributes or characteristics of nurses are the material from which individual nurses make and shape their nursing roles within the constraints identified above. It is beyond the remit of this work to examine the personal characteristics of nurses and their influence upon nursing dying people in any systematic and detailed manner. The two characteristics to be considered here are fear and anxiety, and gender identity. Communication skills will be considered in the following section.

It has been suggested that personal fear of death is related to anxiety about dealing with dying among health care professionals (Glaser and Strauss 1965; Howells and Field 1982; Intermed 1976; Sundin *et al*. 1979). For example, a significant number of the graduate nurses in Gow's study (1982) reported that they were incapacitated from helping dying patients by their own fear of death. A number of studies indicate that such anxiety can be reduced by a variety of educational strategies (Benoliel 1983; Field 1986). Fear and anxiety are, as would be expected, negatively associated with nurses' ability to tolerate an open awareness context in nursing dying people (Glaser and Strauss 1965), and are also negatively related to self-confidence and satisfaction from nursing dying people (Intermed 1976). Individual experiences of death, particularly the first experience of nursing a dying patient, are also known to be important (Hoelter and Hoelter 1980–1; Quint 1967). Thus, improving the first experience of nursing a dying patient through better support and advice is an obvious and essential step towards enabling nurses to cope. From the evidence presented earlier it would seem that one way to reduce anxiety is to provide a positive experience within a supportive work environment, so that these initial apprehensions can be overcome before they become part of a negative feedback sequence of anxiety, avoidance, low satisfaction and reward, and lack of confidence in the nurse's capacity to relate to people who are dying. The literature on ward climate referred to above suggests the type of environment in which this sort of positive learning is likely to occur.

In Chapter two the point was made that nursing is predominantly a female occupation, and a number of consequences of this were identified. In the interviews with nurses no difference between the attitudes of female and male nurses towards their work with dying patients was discernible, although other studies have reported gender differences such as the greater ability of male nurses to cope with nursing dying patients (Intermed 1976). The precise consequences of the female basis of nursing for the care of dying patients are difficult to establish. One important connection is to the 'emotional labour' which forms such an important part of this work (James 1986, 1989). Her analysis suggests that they are connected to the downgrading and invisibility of the care dimension of nursing. She writes,

> Informal caring, nurturing and loving roles, which were a substantial part of the lives of the nurses outside the unit were drawn upon . . . Caring for the dying embodies all these aspects, although they are usually explained in less elevated, more human terms. (1986:186)

Because this type of care is thought to be part of the 'natural' behaviour of women it is felt that it does not need to be taught. It is not closely monitored, and thus it is vulnerable to erosion under the pressure of heavy medical workloads. When nurses are experiencing difficulty in relating to dying patients they may ignore such psycho-social care work and concentrate exclusively upon the highly visible (and essential) bodily comfort work of symptom relief and the like. In this way, to use James's description, the 'love' part of the work of caring for people who are dying is lost.

COMMUNICATION SKILLS

The literature on communication with terminally ill patients emphasizes two main points: communication influences the quality of the experience of dying, and effective communication among caregivers, patients, and relatives is essential if the experience is to be a positive one. Both verbal and non-verbal communications are important in interactions with patients, and with dying patients in particular the non-verbal channel may be crucial. Nurses should be able to 'read' non-verbal signs of distress, willingness to listen, information seeking, and so on, as well as to control their own signals to the patient. The discrepancy between verbal and non-verbal channels is a major source of unwitting disclosure to dying patients in closed awareness contexts that all is not well. If nurses are to work in a situation where disclosure of a terminal diagnosis is normal practise, they must possess or develop a number of communicative skills. They must be able to recognize the point at which the dying patient is receptive to news of their terminal condition, and be able to recognize the nature and extent of the patient's need for truth. They will need to be able to lead patients to an awareness of their prognoses, and to give them appropriate details about their condition. In doing this they will need to maintain their composure, and to be at ease with the patient. The skill of listening is important. Nurses may need to search out patients' fears and anxieties, and to deal with them in a reassuring manner, for example by answering practical questions about pain relief or domestic arrangements. In this connection they will need to know the common fears and anxieties expressed by dying people (Hinton 1984:231–4). Nursing dying patients who are aware of their condition creates communicative problems for nurses of a different kind to those in a situation of closed awareness, as they have to stage their behaviour in such a way as to create trust and confidence in their patients while managing the ambiguities which remain, such as about time of death.

In their discussion of communication with the terminally ill Nimocks *et al.* (1987) identify 'communicational apprehension' as an important inhibitor of conversation with dying people. Such apprehension has two sources, social and individual. It may flow from the structural features of the work environment, such as the organization of work and disclosure norms which inhibit nurse–patient communication. It may also be a product of the individual characteristics of nurses, such as their attitudes towards dying people or their lack of communicative competence. In the interviews with the nurses it was evident that they possessed varying amounts of expertise and confidence in their communicative skills. Statements offered about deficiencies in communicative skills with dying patients included 'I'm just not very good at all' (EO), 'I'm frightened to say the wrong thing' (SA), and 'My command of the English language isn't the best, so actually putting things over I find quite difficult' (ED). Given the hazards to conversation in both open and closed awareness contexts, such deficiencies may be important inhibitors of interaction with people who are dying.

Communication patterns with dying patients are, however, part of a more specialized pattern within nursing (and medicine) of restricting and limiting communication with patients, and deficiencies in communication are embedded within and sustained by traditional methods of nursing work. Clarke, in her review, reports that nurses do not spend much time with patients in other than task-oriented or superficial conversations (1983). Bond (1982, 1983) reports a similar pattern in her study of communication on cancer wards, and found a pattern of routinization of communication similar to that reported by McIntosh (1977). Quint (1967) suggests that the rules covering conversations with patients are unclear and are not taught but assumed to be part of any nurse's commonsense repertoire. The problem, then, is how to learn the delicate conversational nuances which prolonged contact with people who are dying requires. The research of Quint and others suggests that failing to do this, nurses learn to avoid such talk, and that they need support and help if they are to continue talking to patients who are dying. The examples and strictures of their seniors are largely unsupportive and provide examples of how to avoid and shut off conversations about emotional well-being or psychological reactions rather than how to 'open up', facilitate, and manage them.

The two main ways to rectify the problem of deficient communication skills are education and guided experience. Although formal didactic teaching may be beneficial, experiential learning is reported to be more appropriate (Durlak 1978; Maguire 1983; Miles 1987). At present learning of basic communication skills, and the support for trainees to use them in their ward learning situations, appear to be unsystematic and left to chance in many instances. Good role models are also scarce, although Orton (1981) suggests that most nurses learn good practice from this source.

PATIENT CONTACT

The nature of nurse–patient contact is multifaceted and varying, even between the same nurse and patient at different times. What we have examined in this chapter, then, is not a simple depiction of what actually happens in the contacts between nurses and patients, but what emerges from the nurses' accounts as being influential in shaping such interaction, what they believe should happen in their nursing care of dying patients, and how to facilitate this desired type of contact. The discussion so far has indicated that the nature of the work site within which nursing work with dying people occurs sets certain parameters to such nursing work, and that constraints may arise from the methods whereby nursing work is organized, although there may be facilitative and supportive aspects to this also. Together these two sets of variables provide the skeletal framework of obligations and expectations within which nurses will interpret and construct their nursing work with dying patients. Key figures within work settings are doctors and ward Sisters or charge nurses. The attitudes and predispositions of the various participants, in particular attitudes towards death and dying, and towards the disclosure of diagnosis and prognosis to the terminally ill, will also influence and steer nursing work and behaviour.

Nursing the long-term terminally ill is reported by the majority of the nurses interviewed to be easier for them if the dying patient is aware of his or her prognosis (Glaser and Strauss (1965) also found that many of their nurses preferred openness). The open awareness context is for them associated with greater ease in interaction with the patient. The time dimension is important in two ways: with long-term patients the nurse can get to know the patient better, which leads to easier interaction. It is also easier to lead the patient to an awareness of his or her dying over a period of time. In settings like coronary care the high nurse-to-patient ratio may allow such developments to occur over a fairly short time span. Despite their expressed preference for disclosure and openness when nursing dying patients, most nurses seemed to rely on more skilled senior colleagues to actually break the news or to lead patients to a realization of their terminal condition. For most nurses, then, their preferences are not acted upon without facilitation by others. Not all nurses held an unequivocal commitment to open awareness, and these nurses seem to be more typical of the wider profession. For such nurses the nature and organization of their work may be the key determinants of whether or not they nurse people who are dying in an open awareness context. Whether or not a nurse favours such situations seems to be closely associated with his or her experiences of the personal costs and rewards of nursing dying patients. This is best examined by a consideration of the nurse's emotional involvement with patients.

EMOTIONAL INVOLVEMENT

Two contrasting attitudes towards involvement of nurses with their dying patients have been reported. At one extreme, as found on Ward 7, nurses avoid involvement and feel that they should not get over-involved with patients. The student and pupil nurses interviewed on Ward 6 reported that this was what they had been taught in nursing school. By contrast, the experienced nurses on Ward 6 reported that they did become involved with the dying patients they nursed and saw this as largely unproblematic, inevitable, and rewarding. Nurses on the CCU and community nurses fell between these extremes in their attitudes towards involvement with patients. Hockey (1979) identifies conflict between 'professional distance' and personal involvement as one of the central problems for nurses in the care of the terminally ill, while Gow, in her study of *How Nurses' Emotions Affect Patient Care* (1982) argues that emotional involvement of nurses with patients is difficult to avoid, and that attempting to do so in order to maintain professional distance causes problems for nurses, patients, and relatives. Her view is supported by the finding of a large-scale unselective US study that uninvolved nurses were more likely to become discouraged and depressed, and were less confident about their provision of technical and psychological care of the terminally ill (Intermed 1976:152). The study also found that many nurses became personally involved with dying patients and grieved at their death. From the accounts of the nurses spoken to by the author it seems that emotional involvement by nurses in this study with dying patients was more likely to be a positive than a negative feature for both nurse and patient.

The importance of involvement by nurses with the dying patients they are caring for is described well by James in her study of hospice nursing:

> Being 'involved' meant making an effort to be friendly and approachable and responding promptly when patients asked for attention, so that the kind of care nurses felt able to give depended on personal factors, their own feelings, as well as on how Byresford was organised. . . .

> 'Care' requires time, involvement, and a good atmosphere, but this is part of getting information about an individual

133

patient which may then be remembered for future use, or
acted upon by all nurses to improve an ill-person's care. . . .
The emotional involvement was part of getting to know the
patients, . . .

(1986:157)

A system of individualized patient care seems to be associated with
good nursing care of those who are dying and, it seems, inevitably
creates a certain amount of involvement. It is clear, however, that
high levels of involvement may cause difficulties for nurses, and
that many nurses therefore endeavour to limit or avoid it. Vachon
reports that overinvolvement with patients is a source of stress for
nurses (1987). If emotional involvement with dying patients is
indeed inevitable under the individualized methods of patient care
which are being promoted by the leadership of the nursing profession, then the problems which such involvement may cause nurses
must be dealt with. The rewarding and beneficial aspects of
emotional involvement which were reported by many of the nurses
interviewed may for some nurses be insufficient on their own to
offset the difficulties engendered. Better training and preparation
may help, but a good and easily available system of social and
psychological support for nurses is an obvious corollary to
individualized patient care. Nursing dying people is not, after all,
the only type of nursing work which creates personal coping
problems for nurses; 'caring for the carers' is essential. As
Charles-Edwards comments,

> the value to the patient of close, trusting relationships has
> been demonstrated repeatedly, and it is essential that this
> should become more widely acknowledged and accepted by
> nurse managers. Only then will they begin to look at the
> emotional needs of nurses created by these relationships and
> seek ways of meeting them. (1983:240)

SOME RECOMMENDATIONS

The preceding discussion suggests a number of ways in which the
care of people who are dying could be improved to the benefit of
both nurses and patients. First, nurses should be allowed greater
autonomy and decision-making capacity in their care of patients.
As the main caregivers, who are in 24-hour contact with patients,

and who articulate and coordinate the work of other hospital staff, nurses are ideally placed to appreciate the psycho-social and physical needs of dying patients. A number of writers have commented that nurses frequently give guidance and advice to doctors concerning patient care, although they must disguise this in such a way that it does not undermine the doctor's authority, and so that it appears that decisions are being made by the doctor (Bond and Bond 1986; Game and Pringle 1983; Salvage 1985). The experience of the coronary care unit and Ward 6 at Midland General supports the view that such dissimulation is unnecessary, and that nurses can exercise autonomy and decision making in patient care to advantage.

Second, nursing work should be organized through individual patient allocation and the use of the nursing process. The first component of this suggestion is the most important element; the nursing process is an adjunct to the continuity of nurse–patient contact. The evidence from Ward 6 in particular suggests that the nurses' belief in the efficacy of the nursing process as a tool for good patient care is central to making it work in this way. Good psycho-social care of dying people and ease in communication between nurses and patients depend upon continuity of contact through time so that nurses can get to know their patients' physical, psychological, and social needs and respond to them. This is difficult, if not impossible, where nursing work is organized along task work lines. Unfortunately, the extent to which patient allocation can be practised depends upon staffing levels which allow satisfactory nurse-to-patient ratios.

Third, an important feature of the apparently successful nursing situations found on the CCU and Ward 6 was that teamwork and support had developed partly due to the low turnover of nursing staff. Hence, greater nurse stability is required to allow teamwork to develop. This can only be achieved by the retention of nurses via better pay and conditions, and the freeing of career advancement from the need to move jobs. Vachon (1987) has emphasized the beneficial nature of team support in buffering the stresses induced by nursing dying people and other work. Such support is less likely to be forthcoming where there are high rates of nursing turnover, for in such situations it is difficult to build and maintain teamwork and support.

Fourth, and specifically related to nursing dying people, wards and units should adopt a clear policy of disclosure of the diagnosis and prognosis of terminal conditions. This policy should be known to all staff, and cases of non-disclosure should be justified. The advantages of disclosure have already been reviewed in the introduction. The difficulty in maintaining most dying patients in a situation of complete ignorance of their terminal prognosis (together with the negative consequences of strained interaction and mistrust, patient anxiety and depression, and the difficulties in symptom management which frequently result from staff attempts to maintain closed awareness) suggest strongly that non-disclosure should be the exception rather than the rule. The importance of full and complete information for all caregivers has also been rehearsed. Disclosure of terminal prognosis does not solve all the difficulties of interaction with someone who is dying, and staff will need to keep each other fully informed on a regular basis, for example at case conferences and ward rounds, of patients' anxieties and what they are being told. If such anxieties are to be alleviated all staff will need to know of them so that they may respond positively.

This leads on to the fifth suggestion, that there should be full communication of information about the terminally ill, joint decision making about their care, and full cooperation within the health care team, especially between doctors and nurses, in the implementation of such care. The centrality of communication to the care of dying patients has been emphasized by many writers, and 'good' communication is essential for a 'good' death experience. 'Goodness' can be defined in terms of 'the extent to which the interactants accept the impending death, receive mutual emotional care and support, mitigate the dying person's discomfort and isolation and complete all "unfinished business"' (Nimocks *et al.* 1987:329).

Sixth, it has frequently been reported that the training of nurses in caring for dying people is less than satisfactory, especially in terms of conversational and communicative skills (Birch 1983; Game and Pringle 1983: Quint 1967; Simpson 1975). Better training and education both in basic communication skills and in death education is needed, particularly of an experiential nature. The first experiences of young nurses should be discussed with them so that they can cope with the death of their patient, learn positively from the experience, and feel that they can cope in the future.

Finally, support services for nurses caring for the terminally ill are poor. Nursing dying people will always involve some nurses in some stress, and will probably be stressful for all nurses at some time during their career. Similarly, nurses will become emotionally involved with some of their dying patients, and so will be vulnerable to grief and loss when they die. Thus the provision of support services, especially for those in particularly stressful settings (e.g. intensive care units), is important. It might be argued that the provision of formal counselling services and the like are too expensive, but if nurses are leaving nursing because they are unable to cope with the stresses arising from nursing dying patients and other work, this may in the long run prove to be more expensive. The experience of oncology wards and hospices show that support for staff is an important feature of good terminal care. Indeed, it seems to be essential.

SUMMARY

This book has attempted to clarify those features which hinder or facilitate the nursing care of dying people by examining the relationship between social structural aspects of hospital work organization and the action of individuals working within them. At the individual level a number of characteristics which militate against ease and openness in caring for dying patients were identified. Nursing staff are generally young, and hence likely to have little direct experience of death and dying prior to their entry into nursing. They are likely to share the apparently widespread hesitancy and uncertainty found in our society about interacting with people who are dying. Hence, better training and support are needed if the nursing care of those dying in our hospitals is to be improved. Young females entering nursing are likely to see their role as doctors' helpers giving personal care to patients, and their lack of autonomy at work will in part be due to their acceptance of medical dominance in the definition of nursing work. Such unquestioned acceptance of doctors' orders may be detrimental to their care of dying patients.

A number of structural aspects which affected the nursing care of dying patients were also identified. In particular the methods used to organize nursing work were seen as of central importance. Nursing remains a very hierarchical occupation, and despite the new 'professional' emphasis in nurse education to encourage initiative and decision making, it seems that trainee nurses are not normally encouraged to question or discuss treatment with their superiors during their training on the wards. In the wards they are still generally expected to remain silent, accept orders, and respond to commands. Where work is organized on a basis of task allocation their capacity to develop expert knowledge of their patients is diminished, and they are unlikely to be able to exercise autonomy in their care of patients. One can see that in such situations nurses are unlikely to develop or be allowed to practise the types of decision-making and communication skills necessary for the good nursing care of the terminally ill. By contrast, where nurses have a high degree of autonomy and where individualized patient care is the norm, as on the medical ward and the CCU, the organization of work seems to encourage – even demand – greater initiative, self-sufficiency, and decision making from the nurses, and serves to support caring attitudes. In such situations the nurse can develop expert knowledge of patients which others will lack, and can therefore contribute meaningfully to the planning and delivery of good patient care.

Chapter Eight

Postscript:
some wider considerations

This book has focused on the interactions between nurses and dying patients. In this final chapter a wider view is taken to consider some important features which affect the possibility of nursing dying people in the holistic way which it has been suggested is most appropriate for their care. The factors which will briefly be discussed are the largely beneficial changes in attitudes towards the care of the dying; the impact of AIDS; current problems within nursing; and changes within the NHS; all of which are seen to have negative consequences for the care of dying people. Finally, it is suggested that the personal needs of patients are largely ignored and that the possibilities for human care of those who are dying are diminished by the current work situations of nurses in NHS hospitals.

CHANGING ATTITUDES TOWARDS
THE CARE OF THE DYING

In the more than two decades since Glaser and Strauss published their seminal work, *Awareness of Dying* (1965), there has been a shift in the attitudes of health care professionals towards the care of dying people. The debates generated by the work of Glaser and Strauss, Saunders, Kubler-Ross, and others about *whether* to disclose a terminal prognosis to a dying patient have been largely superseded by questions about *how* to disclose such a prognosis. True, the situation described by Duff and Hollingshead (1968:303) where 'Each member of the group functioned within a framework of ambiguous definitions of what *might* be done, what *should* be done, what *must* be done' (emphasis in the original) has not altered significantly, but the way of responding to such ambiguity seems to have shifted towards openness with patients and away from the evasion which Duff and Hollingshead and so many other researchers have found. While not all doctors and nurses believe that dying people should be informed of their impending death, 'expert opinion' is certainly to do so. Why has this change occurred?

In large part the change has been consequent upon, or at the very least closely linked with, changes in the practical care of people who are dying. The management of pain and other distressing physical symptoms which dying people experience are now much better understood and are more likely to be successfully treated, and so doctors and nurses can now feel that they can offer something positive to their dying patients. Research reported by Parkes (1985) and Wilkes (1984) suggests that a least some British hospitals are achieving levels of pain relief found in the hospices. This is not to deny that there are still major deficits, or that too many people die in unnecessary pain and unrelieved suffering, especially those dying at home. Still, the possibility exists, and is *known* to exist, for the relief of physical distress. It is also recognized that the control and relief of such physical symptoms as pain and breathlessness contribute significantly to the alleviation and reduction of anxiety, depression, and psychological distress among those who are dying. These changes in technology and in knowledge, by providing the means for better physical care of dying patients and a better understanding of how to manage the process of dying, have been important factors leading to greater openness with the terminally ill. Equally important is that many doctors and nurses are no longer seeing death as a failure (Wilkes 1986). The development and dissemination of such attitudes, expertise, and knowledge have been largely a product of the hospice movement which has demonstrated the possibility of holistic patient-centred care, which treats dying people with dignity and involves both them and all those caring for them in the decisions which are made about their care.

Changes in medical and nurse education may also have been consequential in the changing attitudes towards the care of dying patients. In Britain one of the results of the Royal Commission on Medical Education (1968) was the introduction of behavioural science teaching into most British medical schools. In nursing schools such teaching has a longer, better established, and more accepted role. Thus, the present generation of doctors and nurses is more firmly grounded in basic human sciences than previous generations were. They are likely to be exposed to teaching about communication skills, the effect of cultural differences on health and illness behaviour, practitioner–client relationships, and other topics which are relevant to the practice and appreciation of 'whole person' care. In particular nurse education incorporates such an approach as a core feature of nursing practice. They are also likely to receive direct teaching about death, dying, and bereavement, and about their role in caring for those who are dying and their relatives. Despite the acknowledged deficiencies, not least the discrepancy between what is taught in the nursing school and what the trainee experiences and observes on the wards, it seems likely that such changes have led to some changes in attitudes among health professionals and to a greater likelihood of the disclosure of a terminal prognosis to the dying person with probable improvements in care as a result.

THE IMPACT OF AIDS

The importance of nurses' attitudes towards those they care for is clearly shown by the current concerns and fears among nurses about the treatment of patients with Acquired Immune Deficiency Syndrome (AIDS). The rapid rise in the number of people suffering from AIDS poses particular problems for nurses, who are the group of health care workers most closely involved in their care. People with AIDS tend to be young adults – a category of terminally ill patients whom nurses find particularly distressing to care for. They are also likely to be members of two stigmatized groups in our society: homosexuals and drug addicts. There is currently no known cure for or immunization against AIDS, and the death rate of AIDS patients is very high. AIDS patients are thus likely to constitute a particularly problematic category of terminally ill patients whom nurses are likely to perceive as difficult, dangerous, and unrewarding to care for. Reports from both Britain and the United States indicate that some nurses and doctors are refusing to care for people with AIDS either because of fear of contagion or moral repugnance (Shulman and Mantel 1988; Searle 1987; Van Servellen et al. 1988; Zugen 1987). Although most of the evidence about the attitudes of nurses towards AIDS patients comes from methodologically unsophisticated and generally small-scale studies or individual accounts by nurses, a number of themes recur.

A number of reports have come from California, where AIDS is more widespread than in most other areas. Van Servellen *et al.* (1988) in their postal survey of over 1,000 Californian nurses found that the majority of their respondents had a sound knowledge of the high-risk groups for AIDS, and of the precautions necessary for nursing AIDS patients safely. A quarter of them felt that they had a high or moderate risk of contracting AIDS as a result of their work. Slightly under a quarter reported that they would refuse to care for AIDS patients, and a further 16 per cent were very reluctant to do so. Thirty-eight per cent of the nurses reported high or moderate discomfort in caring for homosexual patients. Blumenfeld *et al.* (1987) report similar findings from their study of nurses in Westchester County in 1983 and 1984. One-half to one-quarter of these nurses were fearful of caring for homosexual males because of the perceived threat of AIDS, and half of them said that they would ask for a transfer if they had to care for AIDS patients on a regular basis. Two-thirds reported that some of their family and friends were concerned about associating with hospital staff who had contact with AIDS patients. Geiss and Fuller (1985) in a study of the reaction of hospice staff to their first (homosexual) AIDS patients report that contacts with AIDS patients caused problems for the staff by threatening the non-judgemental stance which many of them adopted towards the values and beliefs of their patients, and by challenging their professional and caring roles. One solution to such problems adopted by the staff was avoidance of the AIDS patients even though this ran counter to the hospice philosophy. Geiss and Fuller identify three issues, which run throughout the literature reviewed: fear of contagion, unresolved feelings about homosexuality (homophobia), and embarrassment by staff about their irrational responses to the patient.

The nursing care of terminally ill AIDS patients thus poses additional challenges and difficulties for nurses. In particular, the fear of death may assume the status of a very real and direct threat for the nurse caring for an AIDS patient. Thus clear procedures to prevent contagion, and in-service and nursing school training about the actual threat of contagion and ways to minimize it, are necessary to alleviate such fears. Given the high level of stress associated with nursing AIDS patients, homophobia and other negative attitudes towards AIDS patients, and the moral dilemmas surrounding their care, staff support and counselling also seem to be high priorities (Geiss and Fuller 1985). In contrast to the United States, nursing guidelines for the care of AIDS patients have been slow to emerge in Britain. A survey of British nursing schools found that while all of the responding schools provided AIDS-related information in the RGN courses there was a 'low level of commitment to skills training' with 62 per cent of the responding schools reporting no such training (Baldwin and Vidler 1988:38). Half of the schools had no policy regarding the management of AIDS. It is imperative that such guidelines are developed and disseminated speedily.

PROBLEMS WITHIN NURSING

Within nursing there is a trend to increasing technical specialization, increasing hierarchy and division of labour, and widening status differences. These trends seem to be linked to a decline in the Florence Nightingale image of nursing and a newer emphasis on professionalism by the nursing elite and increasing militancy among rank-and-file nurses. These interrelated processes seem to have developed further in Australia and North America than in Britain, but the trend is clearly discernible in Britain, for example, in the recommendations in the UKCC *Project 2000* (1986). Game and Pringle (1983:98–9) note that 'with the proliferation of medical technologies and the setting up of special units, the work has become more *technical* and skilled' and specialist nursing becomes 'hived off' from the general wards, with 'hyperskilling of one side . . . while the other side is deskilled with basic nursing duties devolving to lesser qualified occupational categories'. Such divisions are not particularly new, and have existed since Nightingale introduced her 'lady probationers' into the service, contrasting them to the rough and untrained nurses in the poor house and municiple hospitals of the time. Game and Pringle see the modern pattern of specialization and fragmentation within nursing as eroding traditional nursing values of a domestic and caring kind, and the handing down of such functions to the less qualified, a view also presented by Salvage (1985). What is happening, they claim, is a perpetuation of dependence on largely untrained labour who draw upon the 'natural' domestic skills of being female to carry out the basic nursing care of patients while highly trained and better paid 'professional' nurses work primarily as clinical assistants to doctors. In such circumstances the care of the psychological and basic comfort needs of dying patients are likely to be carried out by nursing auxiliaries while their more complicated clinical care will be handled by nurse specialists despite the undeniably close interrelationship between these aspects of care.

One of the problems for nursing is its peculiar situation of being both independent within its own domain of patient care while at the same time having the scope and content of its work subject to control by doctors (Freidson 1970). Both Game and Pringle (1983) and Salvage (1985) claim that nurses are becoming more independent and are challenging medical authority rather than passively accepting medical control of nursing work. At the level of the occupation, the attempts to specialize and improve entry requirements can be seen as one way in which nursing is attempting to gain more independence from the medical profession. Nevertheless, this seems to have been largely unsuccessful so far, as witnessed by the persistent low pay of nurses despite their advanced preparation and a rising demand for nursing services. A sense of powerlessness and frustration is often voiced among nurses, and a there is a lack of career rewards or advancement for most of them. Under these circumstances it is hard to see where the leverage for autonomy and decision making identified as being vital for the nursing care of dying patients will come from. It remains to be seen what impact the implementation of the Project 2000 proposals will have.

An important problem for nursing resulting from its dependence upon female labour is that in Britain during the 1990s there will be a decline in the number of potential recruits due to the changing demographic structure. By 1997 there will be one-third fewer female school leavers than in 1987 (Department of Employment 1988). Already nursing is in competition with other occupations (e.g. banking) that are seeking to recruit young women to replace their previous dependence on young males, and most alternative jobs in the skilled/semi-professional sectors of the labour market will offer better pay and hours than nursing. Given a difficulty in retaining nursing staff that dates from Victorian times (Abel-Smith 1960; Salvage 1985), nursing faces a difficult time in terms of recruitment and retention of labour, and nursing schools are already experiencing difficulties in recruitment (BBC 1987). One of the disadvantages nurses face in this respect is that, as noted in Chapter two, as they comprise over 40 per cent of the National Health Service wages and salaries bill, the government of the day has a vested interest in restricting their pay rises. With its hierarchical organization, low pay, unsocial hours, and subordination to the medical profession, nursing does not present an attractive occupation to many of today's young women.

The consequence of specialization and fragmentation within nursing, difficulties in recruitment and retention of nurses, and lack of autonomy, respect, and control at work can be seen in a number of ways. Perhaps the most obvious is that beds are being closed because there are no nurses to staff them. The number of part-time and agency nurses working in the NHS has also increased, as has the number of nurses working as agency nurses in addition to their full-time hospital jobs. Thus, for nurses there may be increased levels of stress arising from their work and lower levels of support, with increasing chances of burnout. For patients all of these elements lead to decreasing possibilities of continuity in their care, with negative consequences for the care of those who are dying.

CHANGES IN THE NHS

In common with other advanced industrial societies Britain has been experiencing severe pressures on its health services during the 1980s (Allsop 1984; Hiatt 1987; Rodwin 1984). Advances in medical specialization and high-technology medicine have increased the demands on nursing staff while taking resources away from other hospital departments. At the same time they have been partly responsible for the increasing resource demands upon the NHS. The other main source of increasing demands upon the service is the increasing numbers and proportion of British society who are above the age of 75 (Central Statistical Office 1986). This category is particularly prone to problems of chronic disease and disability with require treatment, and are heavy users of the NHS services (Allsop 1984). A high proportion of the terminally ill will be over the age of 75. The consequence of advances in medical technology and of demographic pressures has been to place severe strains upon the funding and functioning of the NHS. One general response from the British government to such pressures has been a drive for more efficient and cost-effective management of the service. However, despite the impressions given by health economists, it is very difficult to measure health status or the performance of health services in a valid and reliable way, and the types of outcome measures of effectiveness are unlikely to include improved 'quality of life' indices, which are in any case difficult to measure (Dent 1988; Hunt *et al.* 1986), particularly for those who are dying. This drive for efficiency and cost effectiveness has, one suspects, created strong pressures militating against the provision of the 'invisible' and difficult to measure psychological and social aspects of holistic care of dying (or any other) patients.

Another proposed solution is to privatize not only domestic, catering, and laundry functions within hospitals but also elements of patient care. Walker (1984:25) defines privatization as occurring 'when responsibility for a service or a particular aspect of service delivery passes . . . to the private sector and when market criteria, such as profit or ability to pay, are used to ration or distribute benefits and services'. Proposals to introduce private hospitals and specialized units which would both cooperate and compete with NHS hospitals, and to extend private health insurance schemes to supplement health care currently provided by the NHS would diversify the range and type of health care institutions (see, for example, Green 1986). It is difficult to predict the impact of such changes upon the care of dying patients, but they may lead to conflicts between hospitals and specialized units and within hospitals, and introduce even more competition between the different aspects of hospital functioning identified in Chapter two. Wards and units may be placed in direct competition with each other for scarce resources which will be allocated on the basis of narrowly defined productivity measures such as bed occupancy, patient turnover, and cost per patient. On a hospital-wide scale one of the net effects seems likely to be an increase in demand for elective procedures accompanied by an increase in waiting time for unprofitable 'cinderella' services such as geriatric medicine. People dying from long-term chronic conditions are likely to be disadvantaged by such a shift in service emphasis.

The net effect of such pressures and changes is a system which is increasingly preventing nurses from implementing whole patient care by forcing them to attend simply to the physical and clinical aspects of patient treatment. Nurses are overworked, exploited, and unsupported in a system which is generating a high level of demand and stress. If the system is inhumane to the carers, how can the carers offer humane care to their patients?

POWERLESS PATIENTS

The theme of nurse–patient communication has run throughout this book. An enduring aspect of doctor–nurse, nurse–patient, and doctor–patient relationships in each case is the control of the information given to the latter by the former. Many writers have noted the control of information and communication is an important way in which people control others. Sharing knowledge is equivalent to sharing power. Controlling the information they give to nurses is an important way in which doctors maintain their authority and control over them. Game and Pringle (1983) argue that in a similar way nurses maintain control over patients. Withholding information from patients denies them autonomy and makes it impossible for them to break down the hierarchical relations which are the normal pattern within hospitals, and so contributes to the depersonalization of patient care.

An endemic feature of hospital care is the neglect of the patient as a person. Patients are treated as passive receivers of what the experts (i.e. doctors) deem is best for them. Medical expertise is typically focused upon intervention and cure of pathological disease processes and conditions. The experts concentrate on the sub-individual features of symptoms, pathological processes and bodily signs, and apply their sophisticated medical and surgical technology to the treatment of these. Such treatment may often be inappropriate for the care of chronically ill and dying patients, where palliative care is more appropriate. In all this medically defined activity the needs of the patient as a person are often overlooked. Nurses usually accept doctors' definitions of treatment and care and so support this depersonalization of patients. They are more likely to act as advocates and interpreters of the doctor to the patient than vice versa. The widespread failure of hospital staff to provide patients with information about their condition

147

seems firmly rooted in these attitudes towards treatment, despite the evidence suggesting that clinical outcomes can be improved by giving patients routine and simple information about their condition and its treatment (Egbert *et al.* 1964; Korsch and Negrette 1972; Skipper and Leonard 1968). Further, dying patients in hospitals are often denied knowledge about their condition while their relatives *are* told. Not only may this have negative consequences for their symptom management and psychological state and place strains on family relations and communication, but this is also a breach of confidence. There are strong ethical grounds for disclosure of information about their prognosis to people who are dying.

Although the majority of deaths in Britain occur in hospitals, most of the care of dying people occurs in their own homes where they are looked after by their relatives, with admission to hospital coming towards the end of their terminal illness. A number of studies report that the quality of life for terminally ill people being cared for at home is often poor (Bowling and Cartwright 1982; Cartwright *et al.* 1973; Parkes 1985; Wilkes 1984). Admission to hospital usually occurs because the main carer cannot cope with care and/or because of problems of symptom control. Despite the emphasis on encouraging community care in place of hospital care for a whole range of conditions the growth of community nursing services which bear the brunt of expert care of the sick and dying in the community is not keeping pace with the increased demand for services (DHSS 1983). An immediate question, then, is to ask why the care of those who are dying in their own homes – where it seems most people would want to die – cannot be improved. Why should hospitals have become the place where people go to die, particularly as the wards are often too busy to be suitable places for dying patients? Is the poor quality of care at home at least partly a result of patients not being adequately informed about their terminal prognosis, and hence not being fully involved in the decisions which are being made about their care?

The realization of nursing care for the whole person and the derivation of satisfaction an reward from such caring nursing can flow from the types of structural arrangements identified in this work. In particular they seem to be closely associated with individualized methods of allocating patient care. Far from being detrimental to the nurse a certain level of emotional involvement with patients seems to be to the mutual benefit of nurse and patient, and can pertain, as the evidence in Chapter four shows, even in such an apparently negative situation as nursing dying patients. The predisposition to care is, one suspects, an important characteristic of entrants to the health care professions. Studies of medical students suggests that it may quite quickly be transformed as they lose their 'idealism' (Becker and Geer 1958), develop a 'detached concern' (Fox 1957), and in many other ways change their earlier commitment to caring for 'whole people'. A similar process may also affect nurses (Clarke 1978; Melia 1982, 1987). Such change is not inevitable, but structurally induced during the course of nurse training and the early ward experiences as a qualified nurse. It is reinforced by inadequate staffing levels, lack of autonomy and respect in the practice of nursing work, unsocial hours of work, low levels of reward, and lack of support in coping with the stresses associated with nursing dying patients and other nursing work. Vachon (1987) argues that healthy work environments recognize and cater for three major areas of staff need: recognition, support, and enjoyment in their work. The current pressures in the NHS combined with persisting patterns of nursing organization and work seem to make the provision of such healthy work environments within British hospitals unlikely. Unless nurses can work in a humane system which gives them respect and rewards them for humane and holistic patient care, it is unrealistic to expect them consistently to provide such care. If current trends continue the prospects are that their caring labour will become less caring and more labourious, to the detriment of all those concerned.

Methodological appendix

The research section of this book examined the experiences, attitudes, and problems of nurses caring for terminally ill patients primarily through the device of allowing the nurses to speak for themselves. Of course, every nurse had a different biography, a different set of experiences, and a different story to tell, and some were more articulate than others, or more dramatic in their recounting. However, care has been taken to quote from as many nurses as possible, and not to quote extensively from only a few nurses. It will be realized that it has not been possible simply to let the nurses 'tell it as it is'. 'It' is many things. The reality of death, as with any other reality, is characterized by multiple, equally true if sometimes contradictory, aspects, only some of which are responded to by nurses and other participants. In order to bring some shape, consistency, and pattern to the nurses' accounts the author has had to apply his own sense of what is 'being said' by selecting what seems most apt, relevant, and even 'true'. This appendix attempts to provide the reader with some idea of the bases for such editorial work.

THEORETICAL BACKGROUND

The methods used to investigate a research problem are conditioned both by the practical issues surrounding access and resources and by the theoretical presuppositions and prejudices of the researcher. Indeed, the latter also influence the choice of the research problem itself. The present study rests firmly on what is widely known within the discipline of sociology as the symbolic interactionist perspective (Blumer 1969; Mead 1934). In particular, it has been heavily influenced by interactionist analyses of hospital life, as can be seen in Chapter two. The central tenet of this position is easily stated: we are human because we talk. Language allows humans to stand outside and apart from the immediate world of activity in ways which are impossible for other animals lacking humanity's symbolic capacity. Unlike other animals humans interact with each other and their physical environment in a symbolic manner. There is no intrinsic meaning to objects in the world, rather their meaning is constructed, transmitted, and negotiated by humans, mainly through the linguistic medium. Language provides a set of shared meanings about the world which serves to coordinate human actions by directing their attention to salient features of situations, and provides the primary mechanism for the development of self-awareness and self-objectification which are prerequisite for human social interaction (Flavell *et al.* 1968; Mead 1934).

Symbolic interaction emphasizes communication as central to understanding social action and focuses on the subjective meanings which people use to interpret their actions. However, such interpretation does not occur independently of the physical and social characteristics of the settings in which behaviour takes place. There are factors such as legal rules governing permissible nursing activities, staffing levels, and patient flow which, as Durkheim (1950) so aptly put it, assume the nature of 'social facts' which place constraints upon nursing activity. Such social facts may, indeed *must*, be interpreted and negotiated by individuals, even if there are limits constraining such interpretations (Blumer 1969; Strauss 1978). It is such activities which interactionists study. Their method of choice is participant observation, which was used in the study reported in Chapter three. However, this was not available to the author because he could not commit the time required for such a method (i.e. at least full nursing shifts) on a regular basis. Instead, unstructured and informal interviews were used in the studies described in Chapters four, five, and six.

Both participant observation and the unstructured interview attempt to be nondirective and responsive to new and unexpected information, although the latter inevitably has a narrower focus of concern and cannot draw on the direct experience of the researcher. In both the researcher learns by asking questions to test leads and hunches derived from previous research contacts, and both attempt to gather detailed descriptive material on the ways in which individuals make sense of their lives without imposing the researcher's concepts or categories upon such descriptions. Unstructured interviews are concerned with the discovery of new information, and together with other 'qualitative methods which use natural language, are best at gaining access to the life-world of other individuals in a short time' (Schwartz and Jacobs 1979:5; see also Field and Morse 1985). Quantitative methods such as the sample survey are based to a large extent on prior knowledge and information about what is to be studied (although not necessarily in a detailed way). When little is known qualitative methods are better for gaining an understanding of people's attitudes and beliefs, and how these influence their behaviour. In using such methods the researcher must suspend belief in the normal and taken for granted assumptions about the social world and its organisation, and instead attempt to discover how the people being studied organize their behaviour and make sense of their world (Hammersley and Atkinson 1983). Such a setting aside of one's day-to-day knowledge is easier in a strange situation than in one which is familiar. It is, however, an essential and important feature of this type of research.

THE SAMPLE

The medical ward and the coronary care unit (CCU) referred to in this study were part of a medium-sized (900-bed) general hospital located in a Midlands city in England. Access to the medical wards and the CCU was obtained through the nursing officer, and nurses were free to refuse being interviewed. The entire day staff (18 nurses) of a general medical ward were interviewed over a nine-week period in 1982. All but two of them were female, and their nursing experience ranged from trainees on their first ward to one nurse with 20 years' experience. Most of the nurses working in the general medical setting (12) were between the ages of 20 and 25. Nine of the ten trainee nurses interviewed for the study were working on Ward 6. Nineteen of the 20 nurses working on the coronary care unit were interviewed over an eight-week period in 1983. One of these was a final-year student nurse and the remainder were all qualified nurses. Eight of the nurses were male. The third group interviewed were qualified nurses taking the District Nurse Certificate course at the city's nursing school. The 14 nurses who had indicated their consent were interviewed towards the end of their course and after lectures had finished during a six-week period in 1984. Eight of these had already worked as community nurses, the remaining six entering the course from hospital work. By the time of interview all of them had experienced at least two deaths of patients they had been nursing in the community. This 'community nurse' group had the oldest mean age of the three interview groups (30.6) with a range of 23 to 54 years.

DATA COLLECTION AND ANALYSIS

Informal audiotaped interviews were conducted with each nurse. These were very variable in duration, lasting from 15 minutes to well over an hour. Interviews with trainees were typically shorter than those with the qualified nurses. All interviews took place away from the main work setting, but adjacent to it in the hospital interviews. The interviews were unstructured and conversational in style and there was no interview schedule, and no prespecified set of questions which *had* to be asked. Although there was an agenda of topics which the author hoped to cover, the emphasis was on allowing the nurse to talk freely and to provide as much detail as possible. After the interview the author transcribed the conversation, which was then typed. A copy of the typed manuscript was sent to the nurse once all the interviews with the group had been completed so that s/he could see what had been said and to allow for any censoring of the transcript, although in fact no one did so. The interviews with the nurses on the CCU were preceded by several visits to the unit to observe what was happening. This was felt to be necessary because the author knew very little about the functioning of coronary care units. Time was also spent in observation (mainly at the nursing station) during the interviewing period. In addition to providing a better sense of the functioning of the unit such observation served to introduce the author to the nurses and other unit staff. It also served to supplement interview material and to provide a way of checking nurses' interview accounts with their behaviour towards patients.

A portable tape recorder was used to tape the interviews because it would otherwise not have been possible to record the nurses' accounts fully. Tape recording greatly reduces the element of selective interpretation by the researcher of what the respondent is saying during the data collection stage (Hammersley and Atkinson 1983). At the start of the interview and before the tape recorder was switched on the author would explain who he was and what he was doing. A typical explanation would be as follows:

> *DF* Basically what I am doing is talking with nurses about their experiences of nursing dying patients. How I got into this is through my teaching at (local school of nursing) where I lecture about death and dying. I thought I ought to find out how nurses viewed nursing dying people by talking to them about their experiences. What I'd like to do is to ask you some general questions and let you talk as much as you want. I probably won't say very much, just let you talk. I am using a tape recorder because that is the best way to get down exactly what you say. After the interview I will transcribe the tape, get it typed up, and send you a copy. That way you can see what you said and can change anything or let me know if you've changed your mind and don't want me to use anything that you've said. You can be as frank as you like because you can always tell me if there is something you don't want me to use. Is that o.k.?

At this point the recorder would be switched on and the interview started. At the end of the interview the nurse was asked not to say anything to other nurses about the questions asked. It should be noted that on the three occasions when nurses indicated that their comments were 'off the record', that section of the interview was obliterated.

In the early part of the interview information was obtained about the nurse's career and her experience with dying patients. The author then asked the nurses from the medical wards if they would tell him about 'anyone [dying patient] in particular you remember', and from that point the interview proceeded in conversational style covering the agenda of topics in no fixed order. Other starting points were used on the CCU and with the community nurse group, which related to their particular type of nursing experience. Many of the topics were introduced spontaneously by the nurse without the author asking about them, and most nurses talked freely with a minimum of prompting. The initial agenda of topics was derived in part from previous research literature (especially Glaser and Strauss 1965, 1967), and in part from ongoing research with medical students (Howells and Field 1982). During the course of the research new topics were added to the agenda as a result of what nurses were saying, while other items were dropped either because all respondents were giving substantially the same responses or because it became apparent that the topics were not relevant to the central concerns of the study. The rationale behind this type of research strategy has been spelt out fully by Glaser and Strauss (1967), Hammersley and Atkinson (1983), and with direct reference to nursing research by Melia (1982).

Each self-contained meaningful statement was coded into as many categories as were applicable. For the author's purposes a 'self-contained meaningful statement' was simply any portion of speech which conveyed at least one intended meaning. These could be single words, such as yes or no, or sentences or clauses (e.g. 'It's much easier to nurse someone who is dying if they know they are dying.'). Large file cards were used to order the categories and to facilitate comparison and cross-referencing of statements. Every statement relating to a category was listed on the appropriate file card and indexed by nurse initials and transcript page number, together with a brief indication of content. An example is shown below:

Specimen file card: Emotional Involvement (Ward 6)

SA	p. 1	Shouldn't get involved; can't help it.
PM	p. 1	Her first death: man with cancer, crippled.
	pp. 4 & 5	Trying to retain distance but can't with nursing process and patient allocation. NOT an advantage to get involved.
PF	p. 4	Gets involved, but no problems tho' affects/upsets her for a DAY.
SG	p. 5	Never been emotionally involved with a patient.

and so on. Each group of nurses was listed separately to allow easy comparison within and between groups. In the process of reading and categorizing the transcripts, and in comparing items

155

within the same category, new agenda topics and categories were generated. As this process continued certain regularities within categories became evident and a category might be judged to be 'theoretically saturated' (Glaser and Strauss 1967), that is no new information was being found. When this happened only a count of the category instance was recorded. Some categories were dropped from the interview agenda and others modified to elicit more precise and useful data as a result of this categorization process. The main categories used can be seen in the tables in Chapters four, five, and six.

GENERAL PROBLEMS OF THE INTERVIEW METHOD

There are a number of problems with the interview method of data collection which have been extensively reviewed (Cicourel 1964; Denzin 1970; Hammersley and Atkinson 1983; Hyman 1954; Schwartz and Jacobs 1979). Cicourel perhaps overstates the case with his remark that 'interviewing is complex and difficult because it necessitates presenting, establishing, and maintaining appropriate and possibly conflicting roles' (1964:76). Nevertheless, his critical reworking of Hyman's seminal work and his list of 'unavoidable problems . . . basic to the interview and routine exchanges in everyday life' (p. 99) aptly identifies and discusses the problems encountered in the present study. His analysis therefore provides the guidelines for the following account.

Cicourel's first set of 'unavoidable problems' is that 'The nature of responses generally depends on trust developed early in the relationship, status differences, differential perception and interpretation placed on questions and responses, the control exercised by the interviewer, and so forth' (p. 99). It is vital to establish trust and rapport with the interviewee in unstructured interviewing because this method of interviewing is particularly vulnerable to breakdown. Also, the topics being studied are often of a sensitive or delicate nature. Generally it seemed that trust was not a problem, as exemplified by the willingness of nurses to talk openly about 'bad behaviour', and to criticize other staff at all levels. They were clearly not always giving 'safe' and 'acceptable' views.

The status of interviewer and interviewee are well known in our society (e.g. through knowledge of media interviews) even by people who have not been interviewed before (Schwartz and

Jacobs 1979). However, other status attributes of the interviewer and interviewee may intrude problematically. Some nurses, especially trainee and enrolled nurses, seemed to defer to the author possibly as a result of his 'latent identity' (Hammersley and Atkinson 1983) of university lecturer, and this may have had an inhibiting effect on their responses. The lack of experience (trainees) and/or their social background seemed to hinder the development of a freely flowing and relaxed interview with some nurses. The language habits and general assumptions of groups (Bernstein 1972; Schatzman and Strauss 1955; Ashton and Field 1976) may sometimes explain some of the difficulties encountered in the interview. As the unstructured interviews depended upon a relatively 'elaborated' mode of discourse, and were attempting to elucidate the underlying bases of the nurse's attitudes, it is scarcely surprising that nurses who habitually used 'restricted' modes of discourse would have difficulty. Although, as Labov has forcefully pointed out (1972), this does *not* mean that such individuals are unaware or unable to express themselves clearly. In such circumstances interviewers need to be very expert in encouraging and allowing people to talk but without guiding their responses. This can be a very delicate balance to maintain.

Differential perception and interpretation need not be a problem. Indeed, the open-ended unstructured interview format is often chosen precisely to allow the expression of a range of perceptions and interpretations. As Garfinkel has observed and documented (1967:77–94), people presume meaning and intent within task-oriented (and other) interactions such as the interview, and their responses reveal the meaning which they intuit. On a number of occasions in my research nurses would interpret a question, comment, or even a gesture, in a way not originally intended and many of these misinterpretations proved to be useful in opening up new areas which had not been previously considered, or in amplifying existing categories. For example, the author had assumed that dying patients were different from other types of patients and initially couched questions in terms of that assumption. A nurse's 'misinterpretation' revealed that this was not necessarily a valid assumption to make, and led to the exploration of ways in which the terminally ill were similar to and different from other types of patients. 'Misinterpretation' and '*naïveté*' by the author were also used as ways of getting nurses to amplify, clarify, or expand on a topic in a non-directive manner, or to cross-check information.

Control of the interview is vital, but must remain unobtrusive, and depends on good interpersonal skills. In my own case interviews were generally relaxed and friendly even though, given the topic, they were sometimes characterized by a high level of emotional affect as well. The move from one agenda topic to the next was generally smooth and part of the natural flow of conversation. As all hospital-based interviews and most district nurse interviews occurred during work time there was an interviewer-perceived time constraint. To a certain extent this restricted the scope of the interviews, although such restriction may well have been a useful focusing constraint. The main consequence was to limit the amount of cross-checking and 'validating' of responses within (but not between) interviews. In any case as Cicourel (1964:99) writes, 'checking out responses for consistency and depth may lead to uneasiness and avoidance patterns on the part of the respondent', which hence threatens rapport and trust.

Cicourel expresses another set of problems as follows. 'Both the respondent and the interviewer will invariably hold meanings in reserve; much remains unstated even though the interviewer may pursue a point explicitly' (Cicourel 1964:99–100). Not only may subjects 'reserve meanings', but the interviewer may also conceal his or her views on matters of direct research interest (e.g. the nursing process) or which might prove to be contentious (e.g. the value of hospices). It may be difficult, yet essential, not to reveal one's own opinions, and to maintain a detached interviewer role while at the same time presenting an involved and attentive persona. While a certain amount of probing may be acceptable it is not always possible to discover all relevant information by way of interviews. Commonly shared meanings and background conditions may be so well known, 'obvious', and taken for granted by the participants that they are not conveyed to the interviewer. For example, although the author was concerned with and enquired about the structure and organization of nursing work it was impossible to assess *all* the changes in working conditions which might affect nurses' responses, and on a follow-up visit to the CCU to discuss the first draft chapter an important amplification about the general context of CCU work during the interview period was obtained. This shows the importance of combining the unstructured interview with other methods of data collection whenever possible.

Conversations are situationally located and so both transient situationally specific features as well as more durable 'universal' aspects were elicited by the unstructured interview. It is important to distinguish these elements from each other, but unfortunately the 'transient elements' are not usually as transparently evident, as in the case of the interview which was interrupted by a cardiac arrest! In this case both parties were distracted by what was occurring in the immediate vicinity to the detriment of the interview. This example highlights a second situationally related problem: the choice of interview site is important, but is not always under the interviewer's control. Interviews conducted in the hospital were subject to interruption, with negative consequences for continuity and 'mood', and one interview was in fact terminated (after 25 minutes) because two interruptions made it too difficult to continue. Situational variables may thus feed back into the control of the interview.

A final set of problems relates to the performance of the interviewer role. Mental alertness and emotional tone may vary with each interview, and these would certainly have some consequence for the interviews and affect the structural problems of interviewer performance:

> the interviewer cannot possibly check his own responses in detail and follow the testing of an hypothesis during an interview; he is forced to make snap judgements, extend inferences, reveal his views, overlook material, and the like . . . the interviewer cannot escape from the difficulties of everyday life interpretations and actions. (Cicourel 1964:100; and see also Hyman's exhaustive discussion, 1954)

In view of these problems we must ask about the validity of using the nurses' accounts as the basis for making statements about the care of dying people. How can one move from verbal accounts to actual behaviour, particularly as we know there is often a large gap between what we say and what we do (Deutscher 1973)? This question cannot be unambiguously answered, and caution must be exercised in interpreting the research reported here. However, there are grounds for believing that the nurses' accounts can be treated with some confidence. Nurses appeared to be frank and open, as exemplified by their willingness to talk about 'bad practices' and to criticize other staff at all levels: they were clearly not giving 'safe' and 'acceptable' views. The interviews have face validity and are characterized by internal consistency and consistency between interviews. Where there is firm research evidence from other sources (e.g. regarding age-related attitudes) the findings are congruent with it. Finally, the interviews seemed to be largely successful in eliciting relevant and valid information – although the interviewer's belief that the interviews are satisfactory and fruitful measures of 'reality' does not guarantee that they are (Hyman 1954). The use of observation provides some sort of 'triangulation' (Denzin 1970) and supports the general picture presented by the interview material.

References

Abel, E.K. (1986) 'The hospice movement: institutionalizing innovation', *International Journal of Health Services* 16:71–85.

Abel-Smith, B. (1960) *A History of the Nursing Profession*, London: Heinemann.

Aitken-Swan, J. and Easson, E.C. (1959) 'Reactions of cancer patients on being told their diagnosis', *British Medical Journal* 1:779–83.

Alexander, J. (1984) 'The organizational foundations of nursing roles: an empirical assessment', *Social Science and Medicine* 18:1045–52.

Allsop, J. (1984) *Health Policy and the National Health Service*, London: Longman.

Aries, P. (1974) *Western Attitudes Towards Death: from the Middle Ages to the Present*, P.M. Ranum (trans.), Baltimore and London: Johns Hopkins University Press.

Armstrong, D. (1983) 'The fabrication of nurse–patient relationships', *Social Science and Medicine* 17:457–60.

Ashton, D.N. and Field, D. (1976) *Young Workers: the Transition from School to Work*, London: Hutchinson.

Atkinson, P. (1981) *The Clinical Experience: the Construction and Reconstruction of Medical Reality*, Farnborough, Hants: Gower.

Backer, B.A., Hannon, N., and Russell, N.A. (1982) *Death and Dying: Individuals and Institutions*, New York: J. Wiley.

Baldwin, S. and Vidler, K. (1988) 'AIDS and general nursing training curricula: a survey of UK schools of nursing', *Nurse Education Today* 8:36–8.

BBC (1987) 'Nursing into the 1990s', Radio 4, April 8.

Becker, H.S. and Geer, B. (1958) 'The fate of idealism in medical schools', *American Sociological Review* 23:50–6.

Bendall, E. (1976) 'Learning for reality', *Journal of Advanced Nursing* 1:3–9.

Benoliel, J.Q. (1983) 'Nursing research on death, dying and terminal illness: development, present state, and prospects', *Annual Review of Nursing Research*, New York: Springer, 1:101–30.

Bernstein, B. (1972) *Class, Codes and Control*, vol. 1, London: Routledge & Kegan Paul.

Birch, J.A. (1983) 'Anxiety and conflict in nurse education', in B.D. Davis (ed.), *Research in Nurse Education*, London: Croom Helm, pp. 26–47.

Blauner, R. (1966) 'Death and social structure', *Psychiatry* 29:378–94.

Blumenfeld, M., Smith, P.J., Milazzo, J., Seropian, S., and Wormser, G.P. (1987) 'Survey of attitudes of nurses working with AIDS patients', *General Hospital Psychiatry* 9:58–63.

Blumer, H. (1969) *Symbolic Interactionism. Perspective and Method*, Englewood Cliffs, NJ: Prentice-Hall.

Bond, J. and Bond, S. (1986) *Sociology and Health Care: an Introduction for Nurses and Other Health Professionals*, Edinburgh: Churchill Livingstone.

Bond, S. (1982) 'Communication in cancer nursing', in M. Cahoon (ed.), *Cancer Nursing*, Edinburgh: Churchill Livingstone, pp. 3–30.

—— (1983) 'Nurses' communication with cancer patients', in J. Wilson-Barnett (ed.), *Nursing Research – Ten Studies in Patient Care*, Chichester: J. Wiley, pp. 57–80.

Bowling, A. and Cartwright, A. (1982) *Life after a Death. A Study of the Elderly Widowed*, London and New York: Tavistock.

Bugen, L.A. (1980) 'Coping: effects of death education', *Omega: Journal of Death and Dying* 11:175–83.

Bullough, V.L. and Bullough, B. (1979) *The Care of the Sick: the Emergence of Modern Nursing*, London: Croom Helm.

Burke, K. (1965) *Permanence and Change*, 2nd revised edn, Indianapolis, IN: Bobbs-Merrill.

Cappon, D. (1959) 'The dying', *Psychiatric Quarterly* 35:466–89.

Carey, R.G. and Posavic, E.J. (1978) 'Attitudes of physicians on disclosing information to and maintaining life for terminal patients', *Omega: Journal of Death and Dying* 9:67–77.

Cartwright, A. (1967) *Human Relations and Hospital Care*, London: Routledge & Kegan Paul.

Cartwright, A., Hockey, L., and Anderson, J.C. (1973) *Life Before Death*, London: Routledge & Kegan Paul.

Central Statistical Office (1986) *Social Trends*, London: HMSO, Table 1.1.

Charles-Edwards, A. (1983) *The Nursing Care of the Dying*, Beaconsfield, Bucks: Beaconsfield.

Cicourel, A.V. (1964) *Method and Measurement in Sociology*, New York: The Free Press.

Clarke, J.M. (1983) 'Nurse–patient communication. An analysis of conversation from surgical wards', in J. Wilson-Barnett (ed.), *Nursing Research – Ten Studies in Patient Care*, Chichester: J. Wiley, pp. 25–56.

Clarke, M. (1978) 'Getting through the work', in R. Dingwall and J. McIntosh (eds), *Readings in the Sociology of Nursing*, Edinburgh, London, and New York: Churchill Livingstone, Chapter 5.

Crow, R. and Kratz, C. (1977) 'The nursing process', Nursing Times Publication.

Culver, C.M. and Gert, B. (1982) 'The definition and criterion of death', in *Philosophy in Medicine, Conceptual and Ethical Issues in Medicine and Psychiatry*, New York and Oxford: Oxford University Press, pp. 179–96.

Davies, C. ed. (1981) *Rewriting Nursing History*, London: Croom Helm.

Davies, C. and Rosser, J. (1986) 'Gendered jobs in the health service: a problem for labour process analysis', in D. Knights and H. Willmott (eds), *Gender and the Labour Process*, London: Gower, pp. 94–116.

Denzin, N.K. (1970) *The Research Act: a Theoretical Introduction to Sociological Methods*, Chicago, IL: Aldine.

Department of Employment (1985) *New Earnings Survey 1970–1984*, London: HMSO.

—— (1988) *Training for Employment*, London: HMSO.

Department of Health and Social Security (1983) *Health Care and Its Costs. The Development of the National Health Service in England*, London: HMSO.

Dent, T. (1988) 'An imprecise science', *Health Services Journal* 98:968–9.

Deutscher, I. (1973) *What We Say/What We Do: Sentiments and Acts*, Glenview, IL: Scott Foresman.

Duff, R.S. and Hollingshead, A.B. (1968) *Sickness and Society*, New York, Evanston, and London: Harper & Row.

Durkheim, E. (1950) *The Rules of Sociological Method*, S.A. Solovay and J.H. Mueller (trans.), Glencoe, IL: The Free Press.

Durlak, J.A. (1978) 'Comparison between experiential and didactic methods of death education', *Omega: Journal of Death and Dying* 9:57–66.

Egbert, L.D., Battit, G.E., Welch, C.E., and Bartlett, M.K. (1964) 'Reduction of post-operative pain by encouragement and instruction of patients', *New England Journal of Medicine* 270:825–7.

Ehrenreich, B. and English, D. (1974) *Witches, Midwives and Nurses*, New York: Feminist Press.

Elias, N. (1985) *The Loneliness of the Dying*, Oxford: Blackwell.

Field, D. (1984) '"We didn't want him to die on his own" – nurses' accounts of nursing dying patients', *Journal of Advanced Nursing* 9:59–70.

—— (1986) 'Formal teaching about death and dying in UK nursing schools', *Nurse Education Today* 6:270–6.

—— (1987) *Opening up awareness: nurses' accounts of nursing the dying*, Ph.D. thesis, University of Leicester.

Field, P.A. and Morse, J.M. (1985) *Nursing Research: the Application of Qualitative Research*, London: Croom Helm.

Fitts, W.T. and Radvin, I.S. (1953) 'What Philadelphian physicians tell patients with cancer', *Journal of the American Medical Association* 153:901–4.

Flavell, J.H., Botkin, P.T., Fry, C.L., Wright, J.W., and Jarvis, P.E. (1968) *The Development of Role-Taking and Communication Skills in Children*, London: J. Wiley.

Fox, R. (1957) 'Training for uncertainty', in R.K. Merton, G.G. Reader, and P.L. Kendall (eds), *The Student Physician*, Cambridge, MA: Harvard University Press.

Freidson, E., ed. (1963) *The Hospital in Modern Society*, New York: The Free Press.

—— (1970) *Profession of Medicine*, New York: Dodd Mead.

Fretwell, J.E. (1980) 'An inquiry into the ward learning environment', Occasional Paper, *Nursing Times* 76 (26):69–75.

Fry, J., Brooks, D., and McColl, I. (1984) *NHS Data Book*, Lancaster: MTP Press.

Gamarnikow, E. (1978) 'Sexual division of labour: the case of nursing', in A. Kuhn and M.A. Wolpe (eds), *Feminism and Materialism*, London: Routledge & Kegan Paul, pp. 96–123.

Game, A. and Pringle, R. (1983) *Gender at Work*, London: Allen & Unwin.

Garfinkel, H. (1967) *Studies in Ethnomethodology*, Englewood Cliffs, NJ: Prentice-Hall.

Garner, L. (1979) *The NHS: Your Money or Your Life*, Harmondsworth, Middlesex: Penguin.

Geiss, S. and Fuller, R.L. (1985) 'The impact of the first gay AIDS patients on hospice staff', *Hospice Journal* 1(3):17–36.

Gilbertsen, V.A. and Wangensteen, O.H. (1961) 'Should the doctor tell the patient the disease is cancer?', in *The Physician and the Total Care of the Cancer Patient*, New York: American Cancer Society, pp. 80–5.

Glaser, B.G. and Strauss, A.L. (1965) *Awareness of Dying*, Chicago, IL: Aldine.

—— (1967) *The Discovery of Grounded Theory: Strategies for Qualitative Research*, Chicago, IL: Aldine.

—— (1968) *Time for Dying*, Chicago, IL: Aldine.

Gorer, G. (1965) *Death, Grief and Mourning*, London: Cresset Press.

Government Statistical Services (1986) *Hospital In-Patient Enquiry, Main Tables, England*, 1984 Series MB4:25, Department of Health and Social Security and Office of Population Censuses and Surveys, London: HMSO.

Gow, K.M. (1982) *How Nurses' Emotions Affect Patient Care*, New York: Springer.

Graham, H. (1983) 'Caring: a labour of love', in J. Finch and D. Groves (eds), *A Labour of Love: Women, Work and Caring*, London: Routledge & Kegan Paul, pp. 13–30.

Green, D.G. (1986) *Challenge to the NHS: a Study of Competition in American Health Care and Lessons for Britain*, London: Institute for Economic Affairs.

Greenwald, H.P. and Nevitt, M.C. (1982) 'Physician attitudes towards communication with cancer patients', *Social Science and Medicine* 16:591–4.

Habenstein, R.W. and Christ, E.A. (1955) *Professionalizers, Traditionalizers, and Utilizers*, Columbia, MO: University of Missouri.

Hale, R.J., Schmidt, R.L., and Leonard, W.M. (1984) 'Social value of the age of the dying patient: systematization, validation and direction', *Sociological Focus* 17:157–73.

Hammersley, M. and Atkinson, P. (1983) *Ethnography: Principles in Practice*, London: Tavistock.

Henderson, V. (1969) *Some Basic Principles of Nursing Care*, Basel: E. Karger.

Hiatt, H.H. (1987) *America's Health in the Balance*, New York: Harper & Row.

Hinton, J. (1963) 'The physical and mental distress of the dying', *Quarterly Journal of Medicine* 32:1–21.

—— (1972) *Dying*, Harmondsworth, Middlesex: Penguin.

—— (1979) 'Comparison of places and policies for terminal care', *The Lancet* January 6, pp. 29–32.

—— (1980) 'Whom do dying patients tell?', *British Medical Journal* 281:1328–30.

—— (1984) 'Coping with terminal illness', in R. Fitzpatrick, J. Hinton, S. Newman, G. Scambler and J. Thompson (eds), *The Experience of Illness*, London: Tavistock, pp. 227–45.

Hochschild, A.R. (1983) *The Managed Heart: Commercialization of Human Feeling*, Berkeley, CA: University of California Press.

Hockey, L. (1976) *Women in Nursing. A Descriptive Study*, London: Hodder & Stoughton.

—— (1979) 'The role of the nurse', in D. Doyle (ed.), *Terminal Care*, Edinburgh: Churchill Livingstone, pp. 42–51.

Hoelter, J.W. and Hoelter, J.A. (1980–81) 'On the interrelationships among exposure to death and dying, fear of death, and anxiety', *Omega: Journal of Death and Dying* 11:241–54.

Howells, K. and Field, D. (1982) 'Fear of death and dying among medical students', *Social Science and Medicine* 16:1421–4.

Hyman, H. (1954) *Interviewing in Social Research*, Chicago and London: University of Chicago.

Hunt, S., McEwen, J., and McKenna, S.P. (1986) *Measuring Health Status*, London: Croom Helm.

Intermed (1976) *Dealing with Death and Dying* (Nursing 77 Books), Jenkintown, PA: Intermed Communications.

James, N. (1983) 'Work: aspects of nursing in a continuing care unit', paper presented at BSA Medical Sociology Conference, York.

—— (1986) *Care and Work in Nursing the Dying*, Ph.D. thesis, University of Aberdeen.

—— (1989) 'Emotional labour', *The Sociological Review* 36 (Forthcoming, February).

Kalish, R.A., and Reynolds, D.K. (1977) 'The role of age in death attitudes', *Death Education* 1:205–30.

Kellehear, A. (1984) 'Are we a "death denying" society? A

sociological review', *Social Science and Medicine* 18:713–23.

Kelly, M. (1982) 'Good and bad patients: a review of the literature and theoretical critique', *Journal of Advanced Nursing* 7:147–56.

Kelly, W.D. and Friesen, S.R. (1950) 'Do cancer patients want to be told?', *Surgery* 27:822–6.

Knight, M. and Field, D. (1981) 'A silent conspiracy: coping with dying cancer patients on an acute surgical ward', *Journal of Advanced Nursing* 6:221–9.

Korsch, B.M. and Negrette, V.F. (1972) 'Doctor–patient communication', *Scientific American* 227:66–72.

Kubler-Ross, E. (1970) *On Death and Dying*, London: Tavistock.

—— (1975) *Death: the Final Stage of Growth*, Englewood Cliffs, NJ: Prentice-Hall.

Labov, W. (1972) 'The logic of non-standard English', in P.P. Giglioli (ed.), *Language and Social Context*, Harmondsworth, Middlesex: Penguin.

Leviton, D. (1978–79) 'Effects of death education on fear of death and attitudes towards death and life', *Omega: Journal of Death and Dying* 9:267–77.

Lowenberg, J.S. (1976) 'Working through feelings around death', in A.M. Earle, N.T. Argondizzo, and A.H. Kutscher (eds), *The Nurse as Care Giver for the Terminal Patient and His Family*, New York: Columbia University Press, 125–45.

McIntosh, J. (1977) *Communication and Awareness in a Cancer Ward*, London: Croom Helm.

McIntosh, J. (1981) 'Communicating with patients in their own home', in W. Bridge and J.M. Clark (eds), *Communication in Nursing*, London: HM&M Publications, pp. 101–14.

McKeown, S. (1980) 'Working in harness: communication and change in two hospital wards', BSc dissertation, Department of Sociology, University of Leicester.

Maguire, P. (1983) 'Doctor–patient skills', in M. Argyle (ed.), *Social Skills and Health*, London: Methuen, pp. 188–213.

Mauksch, H.O. (1966) 'The organizational context of nursing practice', in F. Davis (ed.), *The Nursing Profession: Five Sociological Essays*, New York: J. Wiley, pp. 109–37.

—— (1975) 'The organizational context of dying', in E. Kubler-Ross (ed.), *Death: The Final Stage of Growth*, Englewood Cliffs, NJ: Prentice-Hall.

Mead, G.H. (1934) *Mind, Self, and Society*, Chicago, IL: University of Chicago Press.

Melia, K.M. (1982) '"Tell it as it is" – qualitative methodology and nursing research: understanding the student nurse's world', *Journal of Advanced Nursing* 7:327–35.

—— (1984) 'Student nurses' construction of occupational socialization', *Sociology of Health and Illness* 6:132–51.

—— (1987) *Learning and Working: the Occupational Socialization of Nurses*, London: Tavistock.

Miles, M.S. (1980) 'The effects of a course on death and grief on nurses' attitudes towards dying patients and death', *Death Education* 4:245–60.

Miles, R. (1987) 'Experiential learning in the curriculum', in P. Allan and M. Jolley (eds.), *The Curriculum in Nursing Education*, London: Croom Helm, pp. 85–125.

Moloney, M.M. (1986) *Professionalization of Nursing. Current Issues and Trends*, London: Lippincott.

Morgan, M., Calnan, M., and Manning, N. (1985) *Sociological Approaches to Health and Medicine*, London: Croom Helm.

Munn, B. (1983) 'Communication with patients and family', in J. Robbins (ed.), *Caring for the Dying Patient and the Family*, London: Harper & Row, (Lippincott Nursing Series), pp. 84–100.

Murray, P. (1974) 'Death education and its effect on the death anxiety level of nurses', *Psychological Reports* 35:1250.

Nimocks, M.J.A., Webb, L., and Connell, J.R. (1987) 'Communication and the terminally ill: a theoretical model', *Death Studies* 11:323–44.

Novack, P.H., Plumer, R., Smith, R.L., Ochitill, H., Morrow, G.R., and Bennett, J.M. (1979) 'Changes in physicians' attitudes toward telling the cancer patient', *Journal of the American Medical Association* 242:897–900.

Office of Population Censuses and Surveys (1986a) *Mortality Statistics. Review of the Registrar General on Deaths in England and Wales, 1984*, London: HMSO.

—— (1986b) *Social Trends*, London: HMSO.

Oken, D. (1961) 'What to tell cancer patients', *Journal of the American Medical Association* 175:1120–8.

Olesen, V. and Whitaker, L. (1968) *The Silent Dialogue: a Study in the Social Psychology of Professional Socialization*, San Francisco, CA: Jossey-Bass.

Orton, H.D. (1981) *Ward Learning Climate. A Study of the Ward Sister in Relation to Student Nurse Learning on the Ward*, London: Royal College of Nursing.

Parkes, C.M. (1976) 'Home or hospital? Terminal care as seen by surviving spouses', *Journal of the Royal College of General Practitioners* 28:19–30.

—— (1985) 'Terminal care: home, hospital, or hospice?', *The Lancet* 1:155–7.

Pembrey, S. (1980) *The Ward Sister – Key to Nursing*, London: Royal College of Nursing.

Perrow, C. (1965) 'Hospitals: technology, structure and goals', in J.G. March (ed.) *Handbook of Organizations*, Chicago, IL: Rand McNally.

Quint, J.C. (1967) *The Nurse and the Dying Patient*, New York: Macmillan.

Rea, M.P., Greenspoon, S. and Spilka, B. (1975) 'Physicians and the terminal patient: some selected attitudes and behaviour', *Omega: Journal of Death and Dying* 6:291–302.

Redding, R. (1980) 'Doctors, dyscommunication, and death', *Death Education* 3:371–85.

Redfern, S.J. (1981) *Hospital Sisters. Their Job Attitudes and Occupational Stability*, London: Royal College of Nursing.

Riley, J.W. (1983) 'Dying and the meanings of death: sociological inquiries', *Annual Review of Sociology* 9:191–216.

Rodwin, V.G. (1984) *The Health Planning Predicament: France, Quebec, England and the United States*, Berkeley, CA: University of California Press.

Roemer, M.I. (1977) *Comparative National Policies on Health Care*, New York and Basel: Marcel Dekker.

Rosenthal, C.J., Marshall, V.W., Macpherson, A.B., and French, S.E. (1980) *Nurses, Patients and Families*, London: Croom Helm.

Rosser, J.E. and Maguire, P. (1982) 'Dilemmas in general practice: the care of the cancer patient', *Social Science and Medicine* 16:315–22.

Roth, J.A. (1963) *Timetables: Structuring the Passage of Time in Hospital Treatment and Other Careers*, Indianapolis, IN: Bobbs-Merrill.

Royal College of Nursing (1985) *The Education of Nurses: a New Dispensation (Judge Report)*, London: Royal College of Nursing.

Royal Commission on Medical Education (1968) *Report of the Royal Commission on Medical Education 1965–68 (Todd Report)*, London: HMSO.

Runciman, P.J. (1983) *Ward Sister at Work*, Edinburgh and London: Churchill Livingstone.

Salvage, W. (1985) *The Politics of Nursing*, London: Heinemann.

Saunders, C.M. (1959) *Care of the Dying*, London: Macmillan.

—— ed. (1978) *The Management of Terminal Disease*, London: Edward Arnold.

Saunders, C.M., Summers, D.H., and Teller, N. (1981) *Hospice: The Living Idea*, London: Edward Arnold.

Schatzman, L. and Strauss, A.L. (1955) 'Social class and modes of communication', *American Journal of Sociology* 60:97–107.

Schulman, S. (1972) 'Mother surrogate – after a decade', in E.G. Jaco (ed.), *Patients, Physicians and Illness*, 2nd edn, New York: The Free Press, pp. 233–9.

Schwartz, H. and Jacobs, J. (1979) *Qualitative Sociology: a Method to the Madness*, New York: The Free Press.

Seale, C. (1989) 'What Happens in Hospices: a Review of Research Evidence', *Social Science and Medicine* (forthcoming).

Searle, E.S. (1987) 'Knowledge, attitudes and behaviour of health care professionals in relation to AIDS', *The Lancet* January 3:26–8.

Shulman, L.C. and Mantel, J.E. (1988) 'The AIDS crisis: a United States health care perspective', *Social Science and Medicine* 26:979–88.

Simpson, I.H. (1980) *From Student to Nurse: a Longitudinal Study of Socialization*, Cambridge: Cambridge University Press.

Simpson, M.A. (1975) 'Teaching about death and dying: an inter-disciplinary approach', in R.W. Raven (ed.), *The Dying Patient*, Tunbridge Wells, Kent: Pitman, pp. 92–105.

—— (1979) *Dying, Death and Grief: a Critically Annotated Bibliography and Sourcebook of Thanatology and Terminal Care*, New York: Plenum.

—— (1987) *Dying, Death and Grief: a Critical Bibliography*, Pittsburgh, PA: University of Pittsburgh Press.

Skipper, J. and Leonard, R. (1968) 'Children, stress and hospitalization: a field experiment', *Journal of Health and Social Behaviour* 9:257–87.

Stacey, M. (1985) 'Women and health: the United States and the United Kingdom compared', in E. Lewin and V. Olesen (eds), *Women, Health and Healing, Toward a New Perspective*, New York and London: Tavistock, pp. 270–303.

Still, A. and Todd, C. (1984) *Social Science and Medicine*, 18:667–72, p. 169.

Strauss, A.L. (1970) *Anguish: the Case History of a Dying Trajectory*, San Franciso, CA: Sociology Press.

Strauss, A.L. (1978) *Negotiations: Varieties, Contexts, Processes, and Social Order*, San Francisco, Washington and London: Jossey-Bass.

Strauss, A.L., Fagerhaugh, S., Suczek, B., and Wiener, C. (1985) *Social Organization of Medical Work*, Chicago and London: University of Chicago Press.

Strauss, A.L., Schatzman, L., Bucher, R., Ehrlic, D., and Sabshin, M. (1963) 'The hospital and its negotiated order', in E. Freidson (ed.), *The Hospital in Modern Society*, New York: The Free Press, pp. 147–69.

—— (1964) *Psychiatric Ideologies and Institutions*, New York: The Free Press.

Sudnow, D. (1967) *Passing On: the Social Organization of Dying*, Englewood Cliffs, NJ: Prentice-Hall.

Sundin, R.H., Gaines, W.G., and Knapp, W.B. (1979) 'Attitudes of dental and medical students toward death and dying', *Omega: Journal of Death and Dying* 10:77–85.

Szasz, T.S. and Hollender, M.H. (1956) 'A contribution to the philosophy of medicine: the basic modes of doctor–patient relationship', *Archives of Internal Medicine* 97:582–92.

Tuckett, D. (1976) 'The organization of hospitals', in D. Tuckett (ed.), *An Introduction to Medical Sociology*, London: Tavistock, pp. 225–53.

Twycross, R.G. (1986) 'Hospice care', in R. Spilling (ed.), *Terminal Care at Home*, Oxford: Oxford University Press, pp. 96–112.

—— (1978) 'Relief of pain', in C.M. Saunders (ed.), *The Management of Terminal Illness*, London: Edward Arnold, pp. 65–92.

United Kingdom Central Council (1986) *Project 2000. A New Preparation for Practice*, London: United Kingdom Central Council for Nursing Midwifery and Health Visiting.

Vachon, M.C.S. (1987) *Occupational Stress in Caring for the Critically Ill, the Dying, and the Bereaved*, Washington, DC: Hemisphere.

Van Servellen, G.M., Lewis, C.E., and Leake, B. (1988) 'Nurses' responses to the AIDS crisis: implications for continuing education programs', *Journal of Continuing Education in Nursing* 19:4–8.

Veatch, R.M. (1976) *Death, Dying and the Biological Revolution*, New Haven, CT: Yale University Press.

Walker, A. (1984) 'The political economy of privatization', in J. Le Grand and R. Robinson (eds), *Privatization and the Welfare State*, London: Allen & Unwin, pp. 19–44.

Walker, J.F. (1982) 'Patient–nurse contact in wards of different design', in J.J. Redfern, A.R. Sisson, J.F. Walker, and P.A. Walsh (eds), *Issues in Nursing Research*, London and Basingstoke: Macmillan, pp. 403–41.

Ward, A.W.M. (1974a) 'Terminal care in malignant disease', *Social Science and Medicine* 8:413–20.

—— (1974b) 'Telling the patient', *Journal of the Royal College of General Practitioners* 24:465–8.

Watts, P.R. (1977) 'Evaluation of death attitude change resulting from a death educational instructional unit', *Death Education* 1:187–93.

Webb, M. (1982) 'The labour market', in I. Reid and E. Wormald (eds), *Sex Differences in Britain*, London: Grant McIntyre, pp. 114–74.

Weber, M. (1947) *The Theory of Social and Economic Organization*, London, Edinburgh, and Glasgow: William Hodge & Co.

Wilkes, E. (1965) 'Terminal cancer at home', *The Lancet*, April 10, pp. 799–801.

—— (1980) *Terminal Care: Report of a Working Group*, Standing Medical Advisory Committee.

—— (1984) 'Dying now', *The Lancet*, April 28, pp. 950–2.

—— (1986) 'Terminal care: how can we do better?', *Journal of the Royal College of Physicians of London* 20:216–18.

Williams, R. (1989) *A Protestant Legacy: Coping with Illness, Ageing and Death in Scottish Culture*, Oxford: Oxford University Press (forthcoming).

Witzel, L. (1975) 'Behaviour of the dying patient', *British Medical Journal* 2:81–2.

Zugen, A. (1987) 'Professional responsibilities in the AIDS generation: AIDS on the wards: a residency in medical ethics', *Hastings Center Report* 17(3):16–20.

Index

Abel, E.K. 30–1
Abel-Smith, B. 12, 145
age, and dying 5, 24, 48–50,
    145–6
AIDS 141–3
Aitken-Swan, J. 9
Alexander, J. 19, 119
Allsop, J. 18, 145
analgesia 99, 140
Anderson, J.L. 1
Aries, P. 6
Armstrong, D. 15
'articulation work' 21, 123
Ashton, D.N. 157
Atkinson, P. 22, 152, 155–7
attitudes, toward death and dying
    4–7, 48–50, 127–9, 139–41
autonomy of nurses 17, 123–4,
    134–5
awareness contexts 4, 9, 26–8,
    130–2, 136; CCU 71, 80–6,
    126–7; home nursing 99,
    102–8; medical ward 48, 50–3,
    126–7; surgical ward 37–40,
    43; *see also* disclosure

Backer, B.A. 5, 22, 24
Baldwin, S. 143
Becker, H.S. 149
Bendall, E. 17
Benoliel, J.Q. 116, 128
Bernstein, B. 157
Birch, J.A. 17, 136

Blauner, R. 5
Blumenfeld, M. 142
Blumer, H. 150–1
Bond, J. 28, 135
Bond, S. 7, 28–9, 42, 125, 131,
    135
Bowling, A. 8, 92, 96, 101, 106,
    148
Bugen, L.A. 17
Bullough, V.L. and B. 12

cancer 24, 28–9, 31; on surgical
    ward 35–45
Cappon, D. 9
care 13–14, 22, 121, 129
Carey, R.G. 8–9
Cartwright, A.: analgesia 101;
    care for the dying 1, 3; death
    at home 96, 101, 106, 148;
    death in hospitals 19, 92;
    disclosure 7–9; patients and
    doctors 43
Charles-Edwards, A. 5, 7, 18,
    42, 61, 134
Christ, E.A. 17
Cicourel, A.V. 156, 158–9
Clarke, J.M. 17, 131
Clarke, M. 47, 64, 149
'comfort work' 20–1, 123
communication 111, 136; CCU
    80–6, 122–3; home nursing
    102–8; medical ward 122–3;
    skills 129–31; surgeons 37–8;

surgical ward 42–4; *see also* awareness contexts; disclosure
community nursing 93–8
coronary care unit (CCU), nursing dying patients 24, 63–91, 115, 116, 120–1, 152; awareness 71, 80–6, 126–7; communication 80–6, 122–3; coping with death 78–80; death 70–7; doctor–nurse relationships 75–6; emotional involvement 71, 78–9, 86–7; relatives 87–90; unit 66–70; work organization 63–6, 64–5; *see also* methodology
Crow, R. 14, 17

Davies, C. 12, 13
death: attitudes toward 4–7, 127–9, 139–41; definition of 25; fear of 128; 'social' 25–6; *see also* disclosure of terminal prognosis
Dent, T. 146
Denzin, N.K. 156, 160
Deutscher, I. 159
disclosure of terminal prognosis 7–9, 26, 136; CCU 71, 80–6, 126–7; home nursing 99, 103–8; medical ward 48, 126–7; norms 126–7; surgical ward 37–40; *see also* awareness
doctor–nurse relationships 13–16, 122–4, 126, 144; CCU 75–6; home nursing 94–5, 105–6; medical ward 47–8; surgical ward 41
doctors: and death 78, 116; and patients 43–4
Duff, R.S. 7, 139–40
Duncan, H.D. 111
Durkheim, E. 151
Durlak, J.A. 131
dying: and age 5, 24, 48–50, 145–6; trajectories 25, 50, 72, 88; *see also* death; nursing the dying

Easson, E.C. 9
education, death 17–18, 131
Egbert, L.D. 148
Ehrenreich, B. 12
Elias, N. 6
emotional involvement 133–4; CCU 71, 78–9, 86–7; home nursing 99; medical ward 48–50, 53–7
English, D. 12

'failure', death as 79–80, 116; *see also* coronary care unit
family *see* relatives
fear of death 128
Field, D.: awareness 27, 50; emotional involvement 53; fear of death 128; methodology 155, 157; nurse training 17–18
Field, P.A. 152
Fitts, W.T. 7
Flavell, J.H. 151
Fox, R. 149
Freidson, E. 12–13, 19, 144
Fretwell, J.E. 125
Friesen, S.R. 9, 39
Fry, J. 19
Fuller, R.L. 142–3

Gamarnikow, E. 12, 14
Game, A. 14–15, 17, 135–6, 143–4, 147
Garfinkel, H. 157
Garner, L. 22
Geer, B. 149
Geiss, S. 142–3
general practitioners (GPs) 94–5, 103–6, 108, 116
Gilbertson, V.A. 7, 9
Glaser, B.G., and Strauss, A.L. 4, 139; attitudes toward death 5, 79, 128; awareness 9, 38–9, 44, 51–2, 127, 132; cues to prognosis 38–9; dying trajectories 25, 50, 72;

hospitals 23–4; nurses' work 121; research 155–6; 'sentimental order' 67; 'social' death 25–6
Gorer, G. 6
Gow, K.M. 5, 53, 128, 133
Graham, H. 13–14
Green, D.G. 146
Greenwald, H.P. 8

Habenstein, R.W. 17
Hale, R.J. 24
Hammersley, M. 152, 155–7
heart disease/failulre *see* coronary care unit
Henderson, V. 14, 17
Hiatt, H.H. 4, 145
Hinton, J.: analgesia 101; awareness 8–9, 26–7, 45, 130; death at home and in hospital 23–4, 92, 94, 101
Hochschild, A.R. 120
Hockey, L. 1, 16, 133
Hoelter, J.W. and J.A. 128
Hollender, M.H. 93
Hollingshead, A.B. 7, 139–40
home, nursing dying patients at 92–109, 115–16, 148, 153; awareness and communication 102–8; hospital *vs.* community nursing 93–8; relationships 93–4; relatives 100–1; work 99–102
hospices 29–31
hospitals 18–19; *vs.* community nursing 93–8; and nursing the dying 23–9; as organizations 18–23
Howells, K. 128, 155
Hunt, S. 146
Hyman, H. 156, 159–60

interaction 151–2
Intermed 128–9, 133
interview method 156–60

Jacobs, J. 152, 156

James, N. 12–13, 30–1, 52, 119–21, 129, 133–4

Kalish, R.A. 24
Kellehear, A. 6
Kelly, M. 117
Kelly, W.D. 9, 39
Knight, M. 18, 27, 35, 50, 53
Korsch, B.M. 148
Kratz, C. 14, 17
Kubler-Ross, E. 4, 8–9, 26, 139

Labov, W. 157
Leonard, R. 148
Leviton, D. 17
Lowenberg, J.S. 5

McIntosh, J.: awareness 39, 51, 84; communication 42, 131; disclosure 7, 28–9, 84; hospital organization 24
McKeown, S. 47
Maguire, P. 106, 131
Mantel, J.E. 141
Mauksch, H.O. 19, 24
Mead, G.H. 150–1
medical ward, nursing dying patients on 24, 46–62, 114–15, 120–1, 152–3; awareness 48, 50–3, 126–7; communication 122–3; disclosure 48, 126–7; doctor–nurse relationships 47–8; emotional involvement 48–50, 53–7; relatives 57–60; ward 46–8; work organization 46–7, 60–2
Melia, K.M. 14, 17–18, 22, 126, 149, 155
methodology 150–60; data collection and analysis 153–6; interview method 156–60; sample 152–3; theory 150–2
Miles, M.S. 17
Miles, R. 131
Moloney, M.M. 13, 15, 17, 122
Morgan, M. 20
Morse, J.M. 152

mortality 5, 19, 92
Munn, B. 5
Murray, P. 17

National Health Service (NHS)
  145–7; hospitals 18–19
Negrette, V.F. 148
Nevitt, M.C. 8
Nightingale, Florence 13, 143
Nimocks, M.J.A. 130, 136
Novack, P.H. 8
nursing: attitudes and
  predispositions 127–9;
  communication skills 129–31;
  disclosure 126–7; doctor–nurse
  relationships 13–16, 122–4,
  126, 144; emotional
  involvement 133–4; female
  basis of 13–15, 128–9, 144;
  and medicine 13; organization
  of 12–18, 119–22, 135; patient
  contact 131–2; problems within
  143–5; professionalization
  14–15, 144; recruitment 16,
  145; specialization 20, 143;
  training 17–18, 22–3, 28, 136,
  140–1; ward sister's role 124–6
nursing the dying: AIDS 141–3;
  at home 92–109; CCU 63–91;
  changing attitudes 139–41;
  hospices 29–31; hospitals 23–9;
  medical ward 46–62;
  recommendations 134–7;
  surgical ward 35–45; and work
  organization 113–38

Oken, D. 7
Olesen, V. 22
organization 9–10; CCU 64–5;
  home nursing 96–7; of
  hospitals 18–23; medical ward
  46–7, 60–2; of nursing work
  12–18, 119–22, 135; surgical
  ward 40–1; see also nursing
Orton, H.D. 125, 131

pain 99, 140

Parkes, C.M. 140, 148
patients: characteristics 117; and
  doctors 41, 43–4; nurses'
  contact with 41, 131–2;
  powerlessness 147–9
Pembrey, S. 17, 120
Perrow, C. 20–1
Posavic, E.J. 8–9
powerlessness of patients 147–9
preparation for death 7
Pringle, R. 14–15, 17, 135–6,
  143–4, 147
privatization of health care 146
professionalization of nursing
  14–15, 144

Quint, J.C. 4; age of patient 24;
  attitudes toward death 5, 128;
  awareness 45; communication
  128, 131, 136; doctor–nurse
  relationships 14–15; nurse
  training 22, 28, 43, 136;
  nursing care for the dying 18,
  24

Radvin, I.S. 7
Rea, M.P. 8
recruitment, nursing 16, 145
Redding, R. 5
Redfern, S.J. 16–17
relationships: CCU 75–6; doctor–
  nurse 13–16, 122–4, 126, 144;
  home nursing 93–4; medical
  ward 47–8; surgical ward
  40–2; see also emotional
  involvement
relatives, dealing with: CCU
  87–90; home nursing 100–1;
  medical ward 57–70
Reynolds, D.K. 24
Riley, J.W. 6
Rodwin, V.G. 4, 145
Roemer, M.I. 4
Rosenthal, C.J. 15
Rosser, J. 13
Rosser, J.E. 106
Roth, J.A. 41

Royal College of Nursing 16, 124
Royal Commission on Medical Education (1968) 140
Runciman, P.J. 17, 126

Salvage, W. 13–16, 135, 143–5
Saunders, C.M. 8, 29–30, 48, 139
Schatzman, L. 157
Schulman, S. 13
Schwartz, H. 152, 156
Seale, C. 30–1
Searle, E.S. 141
'sentimental work' 21, 123
Shulman, L.C. 141
Simpson, I.H. 17
Simpson, M.A. 6–7, 18, 42–3, 136
sister, ward 124–6
Skipper, J. 148
sociology, theory 150–2
specialization, nursing 20, 143
Stacey, M. 4, 13
staffing levels 117–18
Still, A. 106
Strauss, A.L.: class and communication 157; hospital goals 19–20, 22; nursing settings 116; nursing work 123; patient characteristics 117; *see also* Glaser, B.G., and Strauss
Sudnow, D. 5, 24–6, 43, 117
Sundin, R.H. 128
support for nurses 137
surgical ward, nursing dying patients on 24, 35–45, 113–14, 116; awareness 37–40, 43; communication 42–4; patient sample 36–7; relationships 40–2; ward 36; work organization 40–1
Szasz, T.S. 93

teamwork 135
terminal care *see* nursing the dying
Todd, C. 106
training, nursing 17–18, 22–3, 28, 136, 140–1
trajectories, dying 25, 50, 72, 88
Tuckett, D. 20–1
Twycross, R. 30, 101

United Kingdom Central Council (UKCC), *Project 2000* 20, 143
United States of America (USA): AIDS 141–2; death education 17; nursing 3–4, 15

Vachon, M.C.S. 5, 9, 116, 123, 134–5, 149
Van Servellen, G.M. 141–2
Veatch, R.M. 25
Vidler, K. 143

Walker, A. 146
Walker, J.F. 118
Wangensteen, O.H. 7, 9
Ward, A.W.M. 7, 101
ward-sister's role 124–6
wards: design of 118; *see also* coronary care unit; medical; surgical
Watts, P.R. 17
Webb, M. 16
Weber, M. 31
Wilkes, E.: analgesia 101, 140; GPs 106; home nursing 31, 92, 101, 148; nurse training 18
Williams, R. 6–7
Witzel, L. 9
women, and nursing 13–15, 128–9, 144
work *see* nursing; organization

Zugen, A. 141